KNOW YOUR HORSE

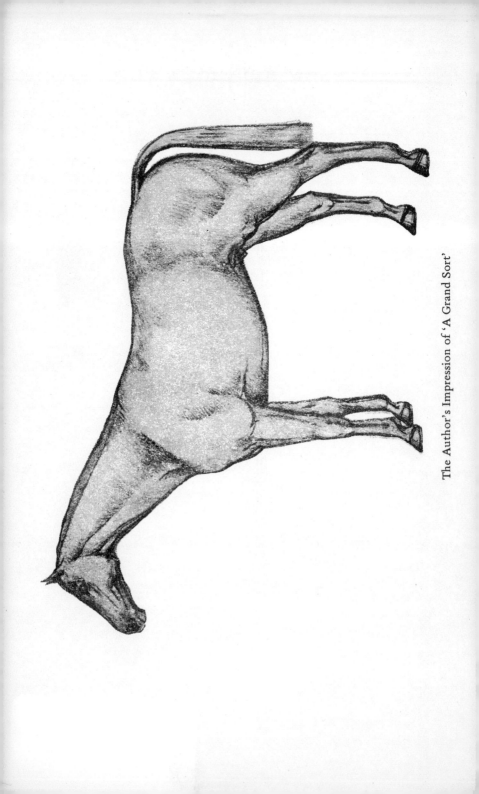

The Author's Impression of 'A Grand Sort'

KNOW
YOUR HORSE

*A guide to selection and care
in health and disease*

BY
Lt. Col. W. S. CODRINGTON
T.D., M.R.C.V.S.

Foreword by Pat Smythe O.B.E.

J. A. ALLEN & CO.
1 LOWER GROSVENOR PLACE · LONDON S.W.1

© W. S. Codrington 1966

First published 1955
by MAX REINHARDT
Reprinted and published
by J. A. ALLEN & CO. *in 1963*
Revised edition 1966
Reprinted 1968
Reprinted 1971
Reprinted 1972
Revised edition 1974
Reprinted 1975
Reprinted 1976
Reprinted 1978
Reprinted 1979
Reprinted 1981

ISBN 0 85131 207 1 Cloth-bound edition
ISBN 0 85131 208 X Paper-bound edition

British Library Cataloguing in Publication Data

Codrington, William Stephen
Know your horse: a guide to selection
and care in health and disease. – 6th ed.
1. Horses – Diseases
I. Title
636.1'089   SF955

ISBN 0 85131 207 1
ISBN 0 85131 208 X   Pbk.

Printed in Great Britain by
Lewis Reprints Limited,
London and Tonbridge

Contents

Illustrations

Foreword

It is my pleasure to write this foreword although I am only a 'layman' in the world of veterinary science. However, as my life is bound up with horses, I am always needing the little veterinary knowledge I have acquired, just as a mother has to deal with the minor ailments of her children.

If I had been able to read Col. Codrington's book before, I could have avoided many of my mistakes. Horses are bound to suffer if one learns how to deal with their troubles only from actual practical experience. This book is a most clear and concise work, covering all the interesting and necessary features so essential for those people who have a concern for horses. It will be a great help to students, but it will be especially useful and intriguing to those interested in the working of a horse not as an organism but as a character that can give pleasure and joy to the rider, and to the people who watch its performance. To appreciate this aspect fully, one must have a knowledge of the basic actions of the horse, and why certain movements are more difficult than others. It is for this reason that I like and value the excellent diagrams of the muscles and limbs.

It is the duty of anyone in charge of a horse to take steps to see that they are able to deal with the many emergencies which may occur and most certainly to be able to render first aid and comfort until professional assistance can be obtained.

This book will also help us to appreciate some of the essential points to look for when buying a horse. Unless one has unlimited funds to spend on unsound horses, it is necessary to be able to recognise those things which may lead to lameness or ill-health, or — to put it simply — how much trouble one is buying with a horse. In fact, anyone who intends to keep or invest in a horse will do well to read, mark and learn these contents. Col. Codrington deserves our thanks, and I am grateful that this book has been given to us from the storehouse of his wonderful experience and success.

PAT SMYTHE

Preface

In presenting a medical treatise to the lay public one must not lose sight of the fact that skill in diagnosis is the main factor in the fight against disease. The script must be in simple language and contain a minimum of technical detail. When the disease has been identified one can, if necessary, refer to one or other of the many excellent text books for the details as to treatment.

Skill in diagnosis is an art, which becomes more polished with experience and one cannot expect that a text book, however comprehensive, will enable a layman to become a Veterinary Surgeon overnight.

In this work I have endeavoured to paint a clinical picture of each condition stressing the symptoms peculiar to it. A diagnostician must observe all the signs and symptoms, eliminate the ones that are common to other conditions and base his final diagnosis on those that are specific. This has been my method of approach.

My conception of a reference book for the lay public is one that strikes a happy medium between technical and practical data, but to do this, it is essential that some knowledge of the normal structure and functions of the body be known, otherwise the suggested treatments may be pointless. Further, I have found that if the cause and pathological processes of the disease or lesion be explained and the reasons for any particular line of treatment be made clear, then the attendant will tackle the case with greater interest and care. After all, what is worse than working in the dark?

For some unaccountable reason some members of the public are averse to accepting any advancement in the world of science, and this applies particularly to the horse world. No one is more conscious than I of the fact that the old experienced hand is very knowledgeable, but his methods and treatments are so often governed by tradition and rule of thumb that anything in the nature of new methods is condemned out of hand. Far be it from me to condemn grandfather's recipes, but I would be relieved if my attempt in this book to enlighten the public as to the value and best use of this venerable old man's tips bears fruit. To the sceptic may I say that science has by no means eliminated the old remedies, but it has offered great aids to diagnosis; e.g. the X-ray in fractures, and given us a number of new remedies, which have specific beneficial action against many diseases.

One final point I would like to stress concerns the tendency of the present day public to make too close a comparison between medical and veterinary science. I am acutely aware of the fact that we owe a great deal to the medical profession for their scientific advancement in knowledge appertaining to disease, and to diagnosis and treatments, and in many cases these things are directly applicable to our patients, but owing to differences in their mode of life, diet, uses and abuses, and lastly, but by no means least, their economic values, there is often a subtle difference.

Lastly, veterinary treatment has to stand up to critical economic standards and this prohibits, in most cases, the full use of many medicinal agents and appliances.

PART I

NORMAL STRUCTURE
AND FUNCTIONS

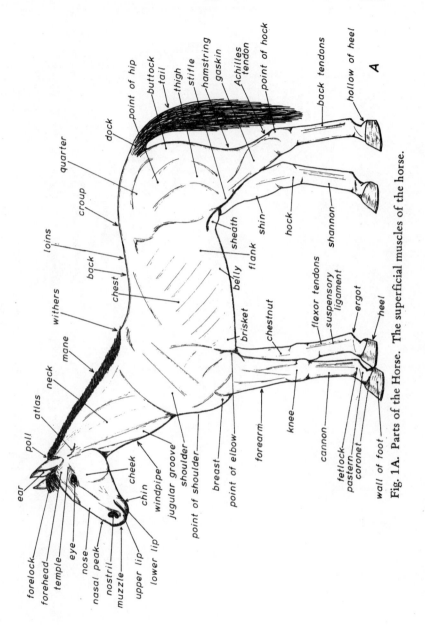

Fig. 1A. Parts of the Horse. The superficial muscles of the horse.

A

forelock
forehead
temple
eye
nose
nasal peak
nostril
muzzle
upper lip
lower lip

ear
poll
atlas
neck
mane

withers
loins
back
chest

croup
quarter
dock

point of hip
buttock
tail
thigh
stifle
hamstring
gaskin
Achilles tendon
point of hock

back tendons
hollow of heel

cheek
chin
windpipe
jugular groove
shoulder
point of shoulder
breast
point of elbow
forearm

knee
cannon
fetlock
pastern
coronet
wall of foot
heel

sheath
belly
flank
shin
hock
shannon

brisket
chestnut
flexor tendons
suspensory ligament
ergot

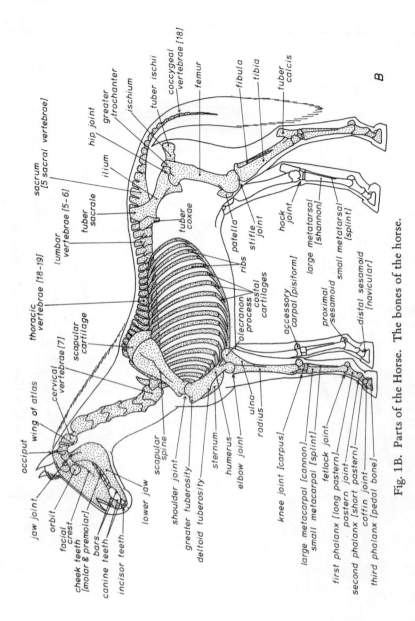

Fig. 1B. Parts of the Horse. The bones of the horse.

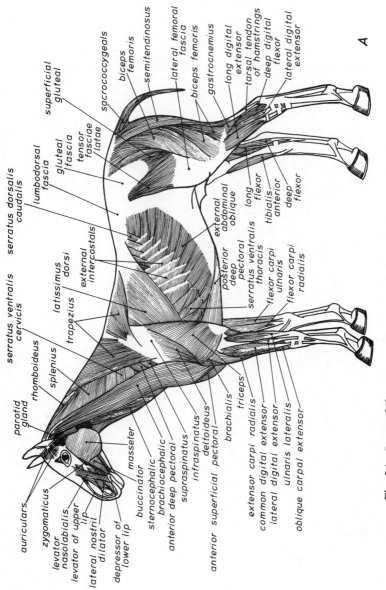

Fig. 2A. Parts of the Horse. The superficial muscles of the horse.

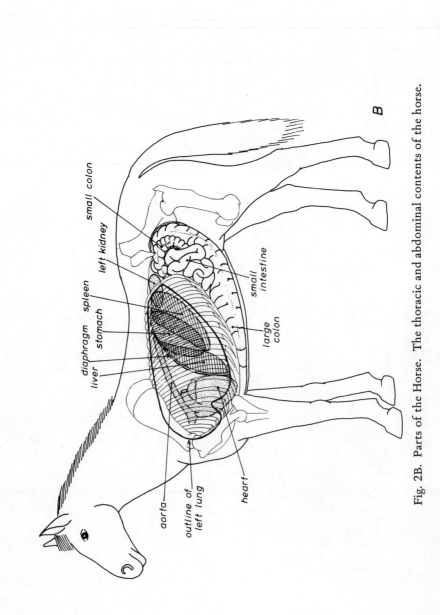

Fig. 2B. Parts of the Horse. The thoracic and abdominal contents of the horse.

CHAPTER ONE

Anatomy

It is obvious that one cannot expect to recognise an abnormal condition in an animal if one is not *au fait* with the normal. Further, to appreciate the normal, other than the clinically obvious, such as a bright eye, good coat, etc., it is essential that one should have some knowledge of the way in which the normal living body functions. With this end in view it is proposed to devote the first part of this book to a simple and brief explanation of the anatomy and functions of the body.

The horse is made up from a head and neck, a trunk, four limbs and a tail. The head and neck form a freely movable mass attached to an almost rigid body. The head contains the brain and the organs of special sensation (eyes, ears and nose) and for efficient usage of these latter organs mobility is necessary. The ability to move the head into a variety of positions is also important from the point of view that it is through the mouth, equipped with teeth and very mobile lips, that the horse 'handles' its environment. The head also provides the passageways for food (through the mouth) and respiratory oxygen (through the nose), the continuations of these channels in the neck being the gullet (oesophagus) and windpipe (trachea) respectively.

The frame is made up of a trunk divided into 2 compartments. The front compartment or chest cavity, formed by the ribs, houses the lungs and heart, while the rear, formed by the abdominal muscles, contains the stomach, bowels, liver, kidneys, bladder, and glands. These cavities are completely separated by a sheet of muscle attached to the ribs and known as the diaphragm.

The underlying basis of the whole body giving it form and support is the skeleton. This is made up of a large number of bones articulated together at joints which are spanned and

1

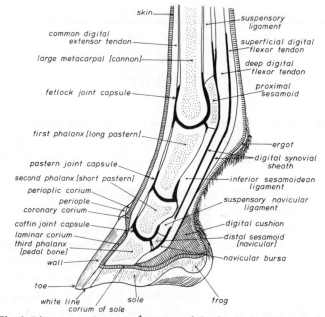

Fig. 3. Diagrammatic vertical section of the forelimb below the knee.

held together by ligaments. For our purposes the most important joints are those of the limbs which are subjected to great concussion. Where two bones meet the joint is made up as follows:

a. The ends of each bone, called the articular surface, are made up of cells which are harder and more dense than the remainder of the bone, to withstand friction.

b. The articular surfaces are each covered by a layer of hard cartilage which is a substance having greater elasticity and compressibility than bone. This resiliency guards against possible bone fracture by absorbing concussion.

c. Ligaments are attached to each bone to hold them together.

d. A membrane, known as the joint capsule, covers the whole joint. This membrane is made up of two layers, the outer being thick and acting as a support to the joint, while the inner layer contains cells which secrete a fluid, known as synovia or joint oil, which lubricates the joint.

Although the skeleton forms the overall basis of the body, posture cannot be maintained and movement will not occur without the presence of a multitude of muscles. Muscles run from one bone to another and so cross joints. They have the power of contraction and will therefore tend to move one bone relative to the other, movement occuring at the joint. Throughout the limbs the muscles are distributed in two major groups depending on whether they flex or extend the limb joints. Flexor muscles bend the joint while the extensor muscles pull it back into position again. However, during standing these same groups of muscles cooperate in a simultaneous contraction to stabilize the joints preventing either flexion or extension.

Each limb muscle is made up from two parts: an upper portion or belly consisting of collections of red muscle fibres which are capable of great contraction; and a lower part or tendon consisting of fibrous connective tissue which attaches the belly of the muscle to the bone and transmits its pull.

All muscles are supplied with nerves emanating either direct from the brain or from the spinal cord. Impulses are transmitted to the muscle via the nerve to bring about contraction of the muscle or group of muscles required to effect a movement.

Because the foot is such an important part of the horse a more detailed description of its structure is necessary.

For the purposes of convenience the parts are divided into a. The skeleton of the foot; b. The sensitive foot; c. The insensitive foot.

The skeleton of the foot is made up of:

The pedal bone (third phalanx or coffin bone) much resembling the hoof in shape but is very much smaller and occupies only a minor portion of the cavity within the hoof.

The Lateral Cartilages These elastic cartilages emanate from the wings of the pedal bone acting as a shock-absorber to the sensitive foot and preserving the elasticity of the foot as a whole. Under certain circumstances they may become ossified the condition being known as 'side bones'.

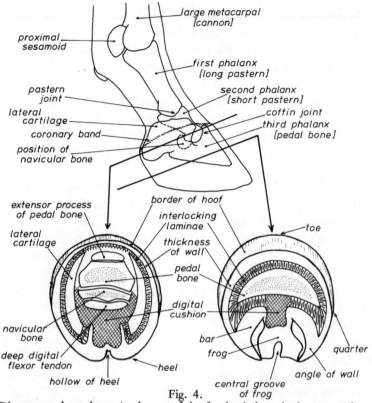

Fig. 4.

Diagram to show the major bones of the foreleg below the knee together with sections of the foot at two levels indicated by the bold lines.

The Pedal (Plantar or Digital) Cushion Lying between the two lateral cartilages is a mass of fibrous elastic tissue situated between the undersurface of the pedal bone and the frog. It has a poor blood supply and is not very sensitive and so it acts as one of the chief shock-absorbing structures of the foot. From above it is pressed on by the tendon of the deep digital flexor muscle when the foot is on the ground and from below it is pressed upwards by the horny frog. It cannot expand forwards to any extent due to the pedal bone and so it expands backwards and sidewards pressing the lateral cartilages outwards which carry with them the horny walls of the heels.

The Navicular Bone This is a small shuttle-shaped bone situated at the back of the pedal bone over which the deep flexor tendon passes before being attached to the pedal bone. It acts as a fulcrum to the tendon.

The sensitive foot is made up of:

The coronary band or cushion encircling the coronet from one heel to the other situated at the junction of the wall and skin which produces horn cells for the growth of the hoof.

The corium of the pedal bone covers its surface and corresponding with the wall of the hoof it is provided with a number (600) of leaves, called the sensitive laminae, which interlock with the insensitive laminae of the hoof wall and hold the pedal bone in suspension. Covering the lower surface of the pedal bone is the sensitive sole, and covering the undersurface of the plantar cushion is the sensitive frog. These three components of the corium are continuous with one another and well supplied with blood vessels and nerves in order to provide nourishment for, and to produce, the horny parts of the wall, sole and frog.

The perioplic ring situated around the hoof head above the coronary band secretes the layer of waterproof varnish which creeps down and covers the wall in order to prevent moisture loss and accompanying shrinkage of the hoof and hardening of the wall.

The insensitive foot or hoof is modified skin composed of practically the same material as the horns and claws of other animals and is made up of:

The Wall is all that part which can be seen when the foot is on the ground. It is composed of dense horn and covered by a membrane that prevents the evaporation of the natural oil. On the inside of the wall are leaves like those of a book which interlock with similar leaves on the sensitive foot. It is somewhat arbitrarily divided into toe, quarters and heels.

The Bars At the heels the wall turns inwards and forwards to form the bars which act as a reinforcement to prevent the wall contracting. The angles at which the walls and bars meet are termed buttresses.

The Sole This is the ground surface of the hoof. It acts as a protection for the foot and by virtue of being convex acts as a shock-absorber. The sole meets the wall at the white line, a layer of softer horn uniting the two. This line is of great importance to the farrier since it indicates the distinction between sensitive and insensitive parts of the foot and the thickness of the wall. It is therefore a guide to the positioning of the nails when shoeing.

The Frog This is the V-shaped structure interposed between the bars. It is made up of a spongy horn and is concerned with the structures inside the hoof in assisting foot circulation.

CHAPTER TWO

Physiology

The Circulation The circulatory system is based upon the heart, a hollow muscular organ situated in the chest cavity. It is actually a pump which sends the blood around the body, in what may be described for our purpose as a closed circuit of pipes. It is divided into four separate compartments and the circulation is described in the following diagram.

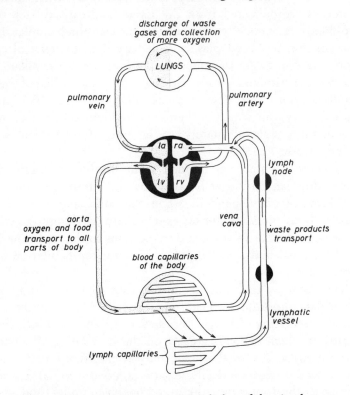

Fig. 5. Diagram showing the general plan of the circulatory system with the heart occupying a central position (la and ra, left and right atria; lv and rv, left and right venticles).

Blood from the right ventricle is conveyed to the lungs where it is oxygenated and then returned to the left atrium from whence it passes into the left ventricle. Blood from the left ventricle is conveyed all over the body in the arteries. Within the tissues the arteries repeatedly branch and decrease in size until they are only visible with the aid of a microscope. These capillaries permit the necessary interchange between the blood and tissues. Capillaries join up eventually to produce veins which convey blood back to the right atrium and thence into the right ventricle.

Complicating this plan is lymph the fluid through whose agency the tissues are directly nourished and by which waste materials are collected from the tissues and carried back to the blood stream. Lymph is a colourless fluid similar in composition to blood plasma and derived in the first place from the blood. At the microscopic level of the capillaries plasma constituents exude through the fine walls of the capillaries into the tissue spaces. The cells are therefore bathed in lymph which is then collected and transported in lymphatic vessels ultimately to be poured back into the blood stream.

Since the lymph has exuded from the blood vessels its circulation can no longer be aided by the pumping action of the heart. It is dependent upon the squeezing action of general body muscles during exercise and the lymph vessels are provided with valves just like the veins so that the flow is unidirectional and space is left behind for the exudation of more lymph.

The return circulation from the foot to the heart is of particular importance. There is a considerable amount of blood circulating through the structures of the foot, the health of which depends greatly on the flow being efficient. The forcing action of the heart and the fact that liquids will run downhill automatically ensure a good arterial blood supply to the foot. Once the blood has given up its food and oxygen to the tissues of the leg and foot it flows into a meshwork of veins encircling the pedal bone and covering the lateral cartilages. In the case of the return circulation, compensation is provided for the uphill flow and absence of the direct force of the heart.

Within the foot, immediately underneath the frog, is the elastic pedal cushion. Each time a horse puts his foot to the ground, pressure from the frog exerts a similar pressure on the cushion which is thrust upwards between the lateral cartilages exerting pressures sufficient to squeeze blood out of the venous network and upwards into the veins on the way back to the heart. To avoid back-flow the larger veins are provided with valves at intervals.

From these details one will appreciate the fact that lack of exercise predisposes to faulty limb circulation — namely filled legs.

Functions of the Blood In the study of disease it is essential that the main functions of the blood be understood in view of the vital part each one plays in maintaining health and combating disease.

The blood is made up of two main parts, liquid and solid.

The liquid, which is known as serum, acts as a vehicle for the solids, and also carries nutritive material in solution from the gut to all parts of the body to aid in tissue growth and repair. It is also the vehicle by which impurities and waste products are discharged from the body, via the kidneys and skin.

The solid parts can be divided into red blood cells and white blood cells. The red part of the former carries oxygen (in solution) from the lungs to all parts of the body and it returns to the lungs in order to discharge waste gas and absorb more oxygen. The difference in colour of the arterial blood from the venous blood is due to the fact that the compound formed between oxygen and the red matter of the cell is bright red (arterial), and when the oxygen is given off, and the waste gases are absorbed, the blood is dark red (venous).

The white cells of the blood, known as leucocytes, are

concerned mostly with disease. They act as the army of the blood, both in defence and attack, and in diverse ways destroy germs which invade the system. Their importance will be appreciated when dealing with the healing of wounds. The diseases of the blood will be discussed in more detail in the appropriate chapters.

Digestion The digestive system consists of the organs directly concerned with the reception and digestion of the food, its passage through the body and the expulsion of unabsorbed materials. The gut tube is a complex structure extending from the lips to the anus. It consists of mouth, pharynx (throat), oesophagus (gullet), stomach, small intestine and large intestine. Associated with the gut tube are several glandular structures such as salivary glands and the pancreas which produce digestive juices active in the breakdown of ingested food. Finally the liver is a major organ associated with the gut and concerned with the storage, processing and breakdown of numerous foodstuffs. Food is essential to life. It is not ingested normally in a form that can be used by the body, but it has to be converted in stages by the action of numerous juices secreted by the gut and its associated glands until the final product is such that it can be assimilated.

The ingredients of a food may be divided into:
a. Carbohydrate subdivisible into a soluble component (sugars and starches) and a crude fibre component (cellulose);
b. Protein – animal or vegetable;
c. Fats;
d. Salts;
e. Vitamins (these are essential food factors);
f. Water.

The main functions of these components are as follows:
Protein builds up muscular tissue and provides heat and energy.
Fats renew fat tissue and yield energy and heat.

Carbohydrates supply heat and energy.

By nature the horse is a muscular, mobile animal dependent to a great extent on its limbs. Horses are used for work of various types but muscular effort does not require appreciable amounts of protein. The primary source of energy for the performance of muscular work is derived from the breakdown of carbohydrates. The diet should therefore provide sufficient carbohydrate; however, if it is insufficient the body can to some extent compensate by converting protein into carbohydrate which can then be used in the normal way.

The simplest, cheapest and most direct method is to provide a ready carbohydrate source. But a number of enzymes are associated with the process of muscle contraction, and several minerals and some vitamins are intimately associated with these enzymes which are derived from proteins. The nutritional problem is then one of supplying sufficient carbohydrate plus the necessary factors for its utilisation which are associated with protein rich foods. The foods for work are therefore carbohydrates containing a certain amount of protein.

We have suggested that a component of carbohydrates is in the form of a coarse crude fibre. A certain amount of fibre is desirable (10%) to aid in efficient mastication and digestion but if too coarse and the percentage gets too high (20%+) the diet becomes too bulky for the relatively simple gut of the horse. The carbohydrates containing large crude fibre components must increasingly give way to cereal grains as a greater work load is required from the horse. This means that the animals diet must deviate in type more and more from the grassy natural food of the species. Digestive upsets consequently tend to be rather common in hard worked horses.

Water is essential to make good the loss that occurs through salivary and digestive secretions and of the excretions of the skin (sweat) and kidneys (urine). As you all must know lack of water is not tolerated so easily as lack of food and condition deteriorates much more rapidly when a horse is deprived of an adequate water supply. There is little doubt that many intestinal troubles are directly attributable to an insufficiency of water leading to solidity of the ingested food mass. It must be stressed therefore that whenever possible water should be given before the food or not for a couple of hours after feeding. A horse's stomach is in fact quite small and cannot contain a full feed together with a large quantity of water.

Salts, of which Calcium, Magnesium, Phosphorus and common salt are the most important, play an essential part in the maintenance of health and development. Owing to the part it plays in the digestion of protein, if common salt were withheld completely from a diet, death would follow from starvation. Natural foods are inclined to be low in salts and in consequence they should be added to the daily diet.

The following table will show the comparative values of the different foods and will give an indication as to their choice for the class of work required:

Average Composition %

			Dry Matter	Protein	Oil	Carbo- hydrate	Crude Fibre	Salts
Grass	..	..	20.0	5.3	1.1	8.9	2.6	2.1
Hay	..	..	85.7	9.7	2.5	41.0	26.3	6.2
Oats	..	..	86.7	10.3	4.8	58.2	10.3	3.1
Barley	..	..	85.1	10.0	1.5	66.5	4.5	2.6
Maize	..	..	87.0	9.9	4.4	69.2	2.2	1.3
Bran	..	..	87.0	14.7	4.0	52.1	10.3	5.9
Beans	..	..	85.7	25.4	1.5	48.5	7.1	3.2
Linseed	..	..	92.9	24.2	36.5	22.9	5.5	3.8

Without going too deeply into the matter a comparison of the analysis of foods in the foregoing table will explain the following:

a. Hay by itself, being relatively low in soluble carbohydrate but relatively high in crude fibre component, is inadequate for hard or fast work.

b. Oats, being high in protein, are necessary for muscular production; being high in soluble carbohydrates they are necessary for energy but low in crude fibre so being readily digestible and not too bulky.

c. Barley may be interchangeable with oats for slow work, but on account of the higher percentage of carbohydrates it is too fatty on its own for long fast work, e.g. horses in training. It is also slightly too low in crude fibre content and may give rise to digestive disturbances.

d. Maize by itself is not a good food for horses owing to its low crude fibre content. A further point against its too generous use is that it is particularly low in salt and almost devoid of lime.

e. Other than its slight laxative action the value of bran will be appreciated for its high salt content, although low in lime.

f. Beans should be fed only in small quantities owing to their excessively high protein content.

g. Linseed should be fed principally as a laxative to fit horses and only occasionally. In the case of sick horses and those in poor condition it is very useful owing to the high fat content.

When compiling a diet, one should aim at the ideal proportion of these ingredients, viz., Carbohydrate two-thirds, Protein one-sixth, Fat one-sixth. Any appreciable variation from this will be uneconomical and harmful.

One final observation concerns the fact that oats contain a greater amount of toxic material than barley. Where a horse sustains an injury requiring rest it is advisable to cut down or exclude oats from the diet. One of the reasons for this is that during rest elimination of poisonous materials is slowed down. Should the injury be a wound these toxic substances will impair healing. However, where barley is fed the quantity may be cut down during rest, but by no means withheld, even in the case of wounds.

Vitamins These are not tangible ingredients, but we know from research work that they are present in varying amounts in different foods. The most practical way of explaining their action, in these days of mechanisation, is to consider the means by which a motor car works. The petrol (food) can only be converted into power if combusted by a flash from the sparking plug (vitamin). For instance, calcium is needed for bone formation, but although a diet may be abundant in calcium, the body cannot utilise it unless Vitamin D is present. Fortunately, vitamins are present in most fresh foods, but the underlying table shows the richest sources of the better known.

Vitamin	Source	Indication as to Uses
A	Green grass, dried grass, silage, carrots, maize.	Resistance to disease and promotion of growth in the young.
B	Carrots, grass, hay, whole grain, bran, yeast, oil cakes.	Action of bowels and stimulant since they are constituents of enzyme systems which regulate carbohydrate, fat and protein digestion.
C	Grass, green vegetable, seeds, roots, fresh milk.	Useful in the treatment of skin trouble.
D	Cod liver oil, action of sun on oil in coat.	Bone formation.
E	Shot grain, green grass, grass seed.	Anti-sterility element. Prevents muscular dystrophy.
K	Fresh green crops	Preventing haemmorhage due to preserving clotting power of blood.

The fact that a horse can thrive, perform light work and maintain condition on green food alone proves that it contains the necessary ingredients of a balanced diet. However, the bulk required to provide the necessary solid (carbohydrates, fat and protein) for heavy work would be too great even if it were available throughout the year. This problem has been solved by drying, but in the process it has been found that the vitamin values are reduced. These values will be reduced even further by bad harvesting, as vitamins are susceptible to excessive heat and fermentation, and also to an overdose of sun. Kiln drying of grain, forced on the farmer by economics, is another process which destroys vitamins.

Where a diet contains a good class hay, cut young so that the seed is not lost, bran and carrots, an ample supply of most of the vitamins will be present. The specific symptoms of a deficiency of a certain vitamin are too complex to consider in this book, but a study of Vitamin D and feeding oats is, I think, appropriate, especially regarding the feeding of foals and yearlings. Vitamin D is the anti-rachitic principle found in such substances as cod-liver oil and its absence from a diet will cause rickets.

Many years ago, Mrs Mellanby proved that certain cereals, low in calcium (oats), led to faulty bone formation. This has since been found to be due to the fact that oats contain an acid which acts on the calcium of the gut forming an insoluble compound. The addition of Vitamin D in the diet partially corrected this, since this vitamin is necessary for the proper absorption of calcium from the intestine.

On further investigation, Mrs Mellanby, in her work *Diet and Teeth*, found that where salt was added to porridge it nullified the action of this 'anti-calcium' acid and an efficient calcium intake was seen. At first you may not appreciate the significance of this, so I must ask you to consider some practical facts which, to my mind, support these findings.

For many years my Father had more than average success in the show ring with young stock and always produced colts with good strong bone and well developed. At the time many of his colts ran on the Severn Marshes and when we went to them we always noted that after a short time, if we licked our lips, there was a distinct taste of salt. This was understandable seeing that the Severn is a tidal river and in consequence, the pasture was impregnated with salt. Further, even when brought off these marshes our colts were fed on a ration of four parts of oats to one part of crushed barley, and salt was added to all grain feeds.

I think I have made myself quite clear that there is ample evidence that oats, under certain circumstances, have their value as a horse food, but in the case of youngsters especially, one must keep in mind this all important anti-calcifying element. Further, the addition of well-bruised barley (the cuticle of whole grain is too thick and hard to be crushed adequately by the teeth) is of great value.

Before leaving the question of vitamins, it should be mentioned that, accepting the fact that they are essential for life, an excessive supply is unnecessary and in some cases harmful.

Specific symptoms do result from a diet devoid of one or other of the vitamins and sensational and rapid cures occur from the addition of the particular vitamin, but it must be understood that the addition of all the vitamins will not convert a low quality diet into a good one.

At the moment Vitamin B is under intensive study and it is found to consist of many very complex parts. A component called B.12, which has an important bearing on the synthesis of proteins and therefore muscle growth and repair, is assuming considerable prominence in the preparation of race horses, enabling them to digest a greater quantity of food. Based on the fact that storage of food has an adverse effect on vitamin values, a great deal has been written regarding the use of them as an adjunct to the maintenance of health. Further, it is not suggested that one must wait for symptoms of each deficiency before ensuring an adequate supply, but, as stated, well-harvested fodder with the addition of some fresh foods — carrots, roots, chopped grass in small quantities, etc., will provide most of them.

The addition of cod liver oil, rich in Vitamin D, to a youngster's diet will ensure a good intake of calcium, but sunlight is of equal importance. One of the natural sources of Vitamin D is by the action of sunlight on the natural oils of the skin, but here again, excessive sun can have the reverse effect. There is little danger of this happening on animals with a good coat, as the hair deflects the sun's rays.

Elimination One of the main reasons for explaining the

components of the blood, circulation and digestion is to
ensure that the reader is in a position to appreciate the
importance of the process of elimination.

As will be seen from 'Digestion', besides assimilable parts
of any food, there is waste or unusable material in varying
amounts in all food, which has to be eliminated from the
system, and should this process be hampered, ill health will
soon follow. The simplest illustration of this is the immediate
sign of ill health following an uncomplicated constipation.

These poisonous materials and waste products may be
divided into two parts; namely, soluble and insoluble. The
soluble waste products are absorbed into the blood with food
from the gut and are eliminated by the kidneys and skin. The
insoluble waste products are eliminated, with faeces, by the
bowel. It is vital to the maintenance of health to keep all
three of these exit channels working efficiently at all times.
This fact cannot be too greatly stressed.

To a certain extent the functions of the skin and kidneys
in elimination are compensatory. If sweating is restricted, the
kidneys will increase their output: e.g. in cold weather more
urine is passed, and *vice versa*.

Further details regarding elimination will be found under
the following section on 'The Skin'.

The Skin Finally, a short study of the function of the skin is
necessary before tackling the question of disease.

The skin has three main functions:

1. As a protective covering to the underlying tissues.

2. To stabilise body heat.

Heat is generated in the body at all times by muscular
movement, or other activity, and is lost by general irradiation
from the body surface and by evaporation of sweat which
cools the skin surface generally. This sweating takes place the
whole time, but under normal conditions it vaporises as it
arrives at the surface and in consequence is imperceptible.
When there is an increased activity of the system and greater
heat formed within, then blood vessels to the skin surface

expand to radiate heat and also to stimulate the sweat glands to produce a more copious flow of sweat which is perceptible. In a cold atmosphere the blood vessels in the skin contract reducing the amount of blood circulating in the skin and therefore the amount which is exposed to the cooling action of the outside air, while the sweat glands show a great reduction in their output.

The expulsion of sweat from the glands apparently involves the activation of delicate muscle cells surrounding the ducts or pores of the glands. Contraction of the muscles and expulsion of sweat occurs in response to certain chemical substances circulating in the blood.

Under normal conditions a balance of production of heat is maintained; in the horse this balance is maintained best when the body temperature is 101° F. (37—38° C.).

In an abnormal condition, such as an infection in the blood, the increased activity caused by the system's fight against the invader raises the body temperature above the normal level. The skin glands do not respond, hence a rise in temperature in the case of a blood disease.

One of the methods of reducing a temperature in the case of a blood disease was to administer drugs which caused abnormal action of the sweat glands and dilation of their pores to enable the patient to lose body heat.

3. To eliminate waste products in solution with the sweat. This is a very important function, hence the necessity of keeping these channels open to ensure health by means of:

a. Grooming: the massage brings more blood to the skin stimulating sweat production and opening the pores, thereby increasing elimination.

b. Clothing: to avoid the necessity of a decrease in sweat production and a closure of the pores to retain heat where the natural coat has been clipped off.

c. Exercise: the increased activity causes an increase in sweat production, opening of the pores and an acceleration of elimination.

I have stated that the functions of the skin and kidneys in

elimination are, up to a point, compensatory, but it must be understood that this is only partial. This may be appreciated from the following case.

Some years ago a small boy, employed by a travelling circus, was painted all over with gold paint as an advertising stunt and he rode into a town on a horse at the head of the procession. Within two days the boy became very ill and before the real cause of the trouble was appreciated, he died. The cause of death was due to the pores being completely closed and the poisonous materials, which would have been eliminated, were retained in the system setting up a 'self poisoning'.

Finally, may I remind you that the full significance of skin circulation and action of the pores will be appreciated when dealing with abnormal conditions of the skin, such as mud fever, etc.

The Nervous System The brain and spinal cord form the central nervous system which is a most complicated structure but I intend to deal with its functions only, as they have a very great bearing on health and disease.

No movement, function, or sensation can be evidenced without the necessary interpretation of an impulse by the central nervous system.

Every part of the body is supplied by nerves from the brain or the spinal cord, and should this nerve supply be cut off by any means, the part ceases to function. Further, when the body is in a state of fatigue, the nerve impulses are slowed down and weak.

To simplify the explanation of the various functions of these nerves, one can divide them into: *a.* Motor Nerves regulating movement; *b.* Sensory Nerves registering sensation.

Two examples of different types of body functions will now suffice to demonstrate how the nervous system works. **Example 1** A pin or other sharp object is applied to the skin. The animal tries to withdraw its body from the offending impulse.

The sharp object presses on a nerve ending in the skin and the pain impulse is transferred by the sensory nerve to the spinal cord. On arrival the impulse is connected with a motor impulse which is passed out from the spinal cord down the motor nerves to the muscles of the forearm and the foot is snatched from the ground. This is a purely reflex action without any assistance or control from the brain. Meanwhile the brain has received the pain sensation, the mind becomes aware of the injury and if necessary a further impulse goes out to the muscles of the limbs and causes the whole body to be moved away from the initial offending impulse.

Example 2 A sudden movement of an object towards an eye causing the closing of the eyelids as a protection to the eyeball.

The nerves of sight register the danger sign of an object approaching the eye, carry the impulse to the brain, from which emanate impulses innervating the retractor muscles of the eyeball causing the eyeball to be pulled back into its socket and so allowing the nictitating membrane (haw) to flick across the eye. At the same time impulses also pass to the muscles controlling the eyelids, causing them to contract and pull the eyelids over the eyeball.

These two examples concern impulses via nerves controlling voluntary movement. There are, of course, a variety of activities in the body which might be termed automatic and beyond the host's control, but still dependent on nerve impulses.

The smell or sight of food will produce the secretion of saliva.

The contact of food on the walls of the stomach or bowel will cause movement of the latter.

Within the skin atmospheric temperature will influence the state of contraction or dilation of blood vessels and the output of the sweat glands.

With the knowledge that all functions can be effected only by stimulation from a nerve impulse and that the latter will be weak or almost absent in the case of fatigue, good horsemastership and stable management must be directed generally towards the prevention of fatigue, or its immediate relief when present.

A very good example which illustrates my point here concerns the state we all know as 'breaking out'.

Some horses, after hard work, will start sweating when brought back to the stable. They may be dried off and shortly break out again. This condition usually occurs in nervous horses and is the result of general fatigue. Like other nerve impulses, those supplying the muscles which control the pores of the skin are weak, and in consequence the latter remain partly dilated. Because of this excessive sweating occurs, and although massage hastens drying off, the sweating will persist until the animal has been revived, in other words, until normal tone has been established. Rugs and bandages may be used to avoid excessive loss of body heat, but often a stimulant is necessary before the condition is relieved. The most efficient stimulant is nourishment in a readily assimilable form. Glucose is ideal as it is a predigested sugar and calls for no further nervous output to digest it. A pound of glucose in a bucket of warm water on return will invariably cure this tiresome condition.

Antibiotics As its name implies the term antibiotic refers to a substance which is anti-life. The group of substances so named are derived from or produced by living organisms and act mostly by preventing bacteria from feeding and in consequence they die. This action is somewhat different from that of the group of medicaments known as antiseptics. which actually kill organisms.

New products of this group are being discovered frequently and the present list is a most formidable one, but I think we must confine ourselves to the better known, as the actions of many will not concern us.

The antibiotics in general use at the moment are Penicillin, Streptomycin, Aureomycin and Terramycin, which have been of service in the treatment of wounds especially for the avoidance of septicaemia following badly infected wounds or abscesses.

The specific effect of some antibiotics is far too complicated to discuss in this work, but their general action with regard to wound treatment is of more than passing interest.

The advent of antiseptics was a very great stride in the successful treatment of wounds, in that they killed the germs with which they came in contact. However, where the wound was deep, the antiseptic was unable to reach them. Further, because they killed or injured living tissue, not only was healing impaired, but the dead cells provided food for the invading germs.

Lastly, the coagulant effect of antiseptics prevented the free flow of lymph carrying leucocytes, which are the healing cells of the blood. On the other hand antibiotics can be injected into the system to combat infections that have gained access to the blood, some having a specific action on certain germs. Antibiotics also have little or no harmful effects on living tissue and they do not coagulate blood. Thus it will be seen that antibiotics have all the advantages in combating infection of wounds, and none of the disadvantages of antiseptics. However, more modern antiseptics such as the Sulphonamide group (Sulphanilamide, Sulphathiazole, etc.) have proved of great use in wounds infected by bacteria.

The only thing to remember when using an antibiotic such as penicillin, streptomycin, etc., is that antiseptics should not be used at the same time, as the action of the former may be destroyed by the latter. To remove discharge salt and water only should be used.

Finally the advantages of penicillin, streptomycin, aureomycin, terramycin, etc., are far greater than the sulphonamide group as the former are fully active when the wound is contaminated by pus whereas the latter are not so effective.

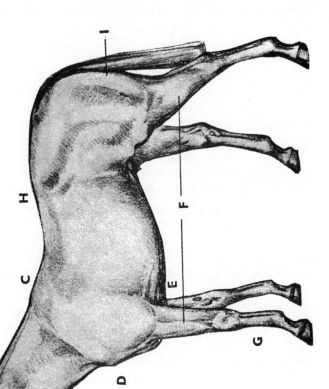

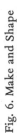

Fig. 6. Make and Shape

A good quality horse with size and substance. The following are his good points:

A.   A good intelligent head and kind eye

B to C.   A tremendous front
C to D.   Good sloping shoulder
C to E.   Deep girth
F.   Good forearm and second thigh
G.   Short cannon bone (knees and hocks close to the ground)
H.   Strong loin
I.   Good deep quarters
C to H.   Nice short back

One fault is that he might be a little strong in the neck, which makes him cresty.

CHAPTER THREE

Make and Shape

Because bad formation predisposes to injury or disease this subject must be considered in any Veterinary work.

Over the years a picture of the perfect horse has been built up, the points being stressed as good because of the class of work required. Naturally there must be some latitude, but in the main, the accepted good or bad points have been proved and they can be dealt with in areas.

Head A good head should be of a size proportionate to the size of the horse itself since an overlarge head may place a strain on the forehand. The muzzle should be well defined with large but not dilated nostrils and the straight faceline should be wide and flat between the eyes. A good width should be present between the branches of the lower jaw. Narrow space will restrict the movement of the throat and might predispose to unsoundness of wind. Thin lips will cover the upper and lower incisor teeth which should meet at the tables. If the lower teeth are behind the upper (parrot mouth) the animal may not be able to graze properly, especially on short keep.

Eyes Large, prominent and clear with uniformly curved lids.

Ears Well placed and alert. Drooping ears are often a sign of sluggishness. Long ears are often associated with speed.

Neck This should be straight and not too heavy since the carriage of the head is largely dependent on the shape of the neck. A ewe neck, especially in a mare, is often a sign of uncertain temperament. The angle at which the head is set on the neck is also important since if too acute there is the possibility of restricting laryngeal movements and therefore breathing.

Shoulders There should be a good slope from the point of the shoulder to the withers. Within reason the greater the slope the more efficient the shock-absorber to the fore limbs.

A further reason, not connected with disease, is that the more upright the shoulder the shorter is the stride, and the horse stands over in front.

Withers Well defined but not too cresty the withers should taper away gently from above to below to provide a wide surface preventing the saddle from sinking down.

Back Seeing that the rider's weight is carried on the back the shorter it is, within reason, the stronger it should be.

Most readers will have heard the term 'a nice short back' but this point is open to considerable argument. Many knowledgeable horsemen prefer a longer back, providing the horse is well ribbed up. This latter term refers to the space between the last rib and the point of the hip. To be well ribbed up this gap should not be more than approximately two inches, a wider gap being referred to as 'slack of a rib'. A study of a number of well-known stayers and winners of the Grand National will reveal a long back in many cases. A likely connection between stayers and long backs may be that a long-backed horse stands over more ground and therefore covers a greater distance with each stride than a short-backed animal. However, the short back can respond to the quick concerted effort required of a sprinter.

Loin and Quarters Since the loin is the least supported part of the whole back it must be as short as possible and it should also be strong as it transmits the propulsive power to the trunk. Strong straight quarters reaching well down into the second thighs, as opposed to rounded quarters, known as appley quarters, are necessary.

Girth and Ribs Long and well-sprung ribs provide a large cavity, which houses the heart and lungs, a good development in both being essential for a sound constitution. In a good horse measurement at the girth exceeds that of height.

Fore Legs The expression 'both legs coming out of the same hole', although an exaggeration, aptly describes a narrow-chested horse and signifies a restricted chest cavity. Further, if the chest is narrow the fore legs will be closer together and more likely to cause brushing. The elbows should be clearly defined and set clear of the body.

Forearms A weak forearm denotes lack of muscle. As some of the muscles in this area activate the principal flexor tendons, a weakness here will mean weak back tendons.

Knees These should be broad and flat to take the weight of the body. Looking from the front, the line of the bone of the forearm and the cannon should be in a straight line, with the knee evenly placed. If the line of these two bones is not continuous, an uneven strain will be put on the knee.

Cannon Should be short and strong with clearly defined tendons behind it. 'Bone' is a term meant to convey the measurement of the cannon region immediately beneath the knee. This measurement incorporates the whole leg, bone and tendons. The term 'a good span' means that the tendons are well developed, as well as the bone.

The term 'tied in below the knee' means weak bone and tendon. As a rough guide a 13.7 horse should have an 8 inch span and a 14 stone and over should have 9 inches.

Over at the knee is the term given to the fore legs when the knee is permanently bent. This is often seen in old horses, as the result of wear, the back tendons becoming contracted, but it may be seen in a young horse and is not a fault. In fact the tendons in such a limb are less likely to be strained.

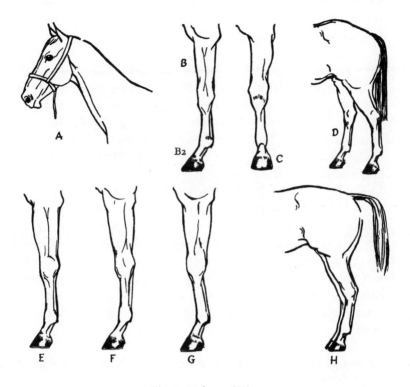

Fig. 7. Make and Shape

A. Ewe neck
B. Weak forearm
B2. Sloping pastern
C. Cannon bone not in line with
   bone above the knee

D. Appley quarters
E. Tied in below the knee
F. Back at the knee
G. Over at the knee
H. Sickle hocks

Back at the Knee This term is applied to a horse whose fore legs show a slightly concave line in front from the forearm to the fetlock joint. This is a bad fault, as undue strain is thrown on the back tendons.

Pasterns A good pastern is set at a gentle angle. The more sloping the pastern, the greater the strain on the suspensory ligament and tendons, thus predisposing to strain of either. If the pastern be upright, concussion effects are not buffered but are registered directly on the joints.

Feet The hoof should be deep with a good width between the heels, known as an 'open foot'. Narrow boxy feet restrict the physiological function of the sensitive structures of the foot and so predispose to disease. The frog should be well developed with a shallow median depression.

Occasionally a horse may have odd-sized feet. In itself this may not be any detriment.

The horn should have a level surface without any marked grooves or rings and no signs of contraction of the quarters.

The colour of the horn is considered by some to be significant, a white horn being weaker than one that is blue or black. There is no direct evidence to support this supposition. Many theories which are founded on experience lack positive scientific proof, but this does not mean that they are erroneous. Col. Codrington always preferred a dark hoof.

Turned in toes When the foot is turned in it is not considered a bad fault and often a horse goes better in deep going.

Turned out toes When the foot is turned out this is considered a very bad fault, as it predisposes to brushing (see Faulty Action), and most cases are unsafe in deep going.

Hind Legs The thighs should be long, well muscled and well let down with no signs of a cut up appearance with a lot of daylight between them when viewed from the rear. The second thigh or gaskin should be strong, as the muscular portion of the tendons, activating the hock and foot, originate in this area.

Hocks These should be more or less square in shape when viewed from the side. If they turn inwards when viewed from the back — cow hocked — it is a sign of weakness, whereas the reverse is often a sign of strength.

If the point of the hock is not well defined, giving the impression that the joint is over-flexed, greater strain will be caused to the 'curb ligament'. These are known as 'sickle hocks'.

A straight hock, the reverse of the former, is often a strong joint. Several celebrated lines of thoroughbred horses, e.g. St. Simon stock, had very straight hocks and gave no trouble in spite of vigorous training.

Cannons, Fetlocks, Pasterns and Feet In each case the same applies as for the forelegs.

CHAPTER FOUR

Description of a Horse

From many points of view it is most useful to know how to describe a horse, either when advertising for sale or during a discussion, and unless the accepted sequence is adopted an accurate picture of the animal will not be gained. The sequence is as follows:

Hunter

Type	Heavy Weight Capable of carrying	14.7	These are
	Middle Weight ,, ,, ,,	13.7	minimum
	Light Weight ,, ,, ,,	12.7	weights

Breeding   Thoroughbred In the Book.

           Hunter   Usually by TB horse out of a good class hunter mare.

           Common horse Usually out of a hunter mare by a light shire or the reverse.

Height   State the approximate height.

Hack   The present day hack is a light weight quality animal, usually in the Book, with good action, about 15 hands to 15.3.

Cob   May be a heavy or light weight, thick set, closely coupled animal. In the past it referred to a short-tailed animal but of course docking is illegal now.

Children's

Pony   This may be any breed and is usually described by stating the height, followed by the words, quality, narrow, stuffy, according to its build.

From the above one can gather the type of animal under

discussion, and this should be followed up by describing the character.

Mouth Good, light, fussy, hard, one-sided.

Manners Good, uncertain, hot.

Movement Free, exceptionally good, poor.

Ride Good, moderate, good in some paces, rough.

In traffic Will pass anything, nervous of heavy vehicles, bad.

The only details remaining to be described are mostly for purposes of identification, the correct sequence being:

Colour Principal colours are black, brown, bay and chestnut.

Sex Mare, Stallion (Entire) or Gelding.

Age If unknown this can be estimated with a considerable degree of accuracy by examining the incisor teeth as described in the next chapter.

Height Calculated in hands allowing 4 inches to the hand.

Markings Such as star, stripe or blaze on the head; flecked or spotted body; white markings on the limbs and variations in hoof colouration.

CHAPTER FIVE

Ageing of a Horse

The ageing of horses is a subject which can be the cause of a great deal of difference of opinion. The argument concerns the teeth and the part they play in estimating the age of a horse. Like any other mammal the horse has two sets of teeth, the first known as temporary or milk teeth, which are replaced by permanent teeth as the animal matures.

According to the position in the jaws they are classified as:

1. Incisor Teeth There are twelve incisor teeth, six in both the bottom and top jaws. The wearing surface has a depression in the centre of the tooth, called the infundibulum, or mark, which disappears gradually with age. The shape of the incisor teeth varies, being oval at the top and gradually becoming triangular towards the root.

2. Canine Teeth, or tusks, two on the upper and two in the lower jaw, appear behind the incisors. Usually they are seen only in the male.

3. Wolf Teeth, two in number, appear just in front of the first molar of the upper jaw. They are minute and have little or no root, and in consequence, are easily removed. There is a popular opinion that these teeth affect eye sight, causing an animal to shy. Their removal is said to cure the habit, but this opinion lacks scientific proof.

Often a horse with a one-sided mouth (a form of evasion) will be cured when these teeth are removed. As these teeth have no value, it is a wise plan to remove them in any case.

4. Molars, six on each side of either jaw, are responsible for the grinding of the food.

For general purposes the front or incisor teeth are the ones under consideration.

The following illustrations should leave no doubt in one's mind how to distinguish between milk teeth and permanent teeth. Fortunately, up to five years of age, the casting of the milk teeth and their replacement by permanents rarely varies. After five years, when all the incisors are permanent, one must rely on other signs, i.e. angles, shape, marks, etc.

These signs are not so accurate as the actual eruption of teeth, but taken together, there should be no real difficulty in estimating the age of most horses to within a year or two.

It is suggested that some animals have softer teeth than others, that a thoroughbred's teeth wear down quicker than those of a half-bred, etc., but after some experience, taking all the *signs* into consideration, this should not affect the average mouth.

Shall we take their ageing in steps, as follows:

1. A 2-year-old shows a full mouth of temporary incisors — six on the top and bottom jaw. Owing to their whiteness and shape there should be no great difficulty in differentiating them from permanent teeth.
2. At 3 years old the central pair of milk incisors are replaced by permanent teeth.
3. At 4 years old the lateral pair of milk teeth are replaced by permanent teeth.
4. At 5 years old the corner pair of milk teeth are replaced by permanent teeth.

Now the horse has a 'permanent' mouth and the other signs must be taken into consideration. The corner teeth having only just erupted, the tops, or tables, will be touching each other at their front ends only.

5. At 6 years old the corner teeth will have worn level. The horse now has the tables of all his incisors level and in wear.

Now one can take stock of further signs, viz.:

a. Cups, infundibula or 'marks', on the tables of the teeth;
b. The shape of the teeth;
c. The presence of Galvayne's groove.

At 7 years old the cup in the table of the central incisors has often grown out but the outline remains. A hook

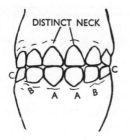
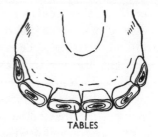

Two Year Old

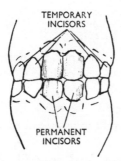
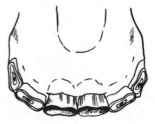

Three Year Old

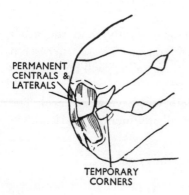
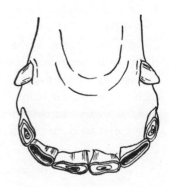

Four Year Old

Fig. 8. Teeth

develops on the back of the upper corner incisor due to it not meeting its opposite number in the lower jaw.

At 8 years old the cup has worn out from the laterals but the outline remains. Between the outline of the cup and the front of the tooth a further mark now appears in the form of a dark line and known as the dental star. It will be seen in the centrals at this age. The 7 year old hook has worn away.

At 9 years old the cups disappear from all the incisors, but the outline will be evident on the corners. The dental star is distinct on the laterals. At about this age a second hook develops on the corner tooth. Unlike the 7 year old hook this is the direct effect of wear.

At 10 years old the cups have gone and the dental star is distinct on all the incisors. The shape of the teeth now changes, the tables becoming more triangular with age.

Another sign to assist ageing appears in the upper corner incisors at 9 to 10 years of age. It is a dark groove and is called Galvayne's groove. It is on the outer surface of the tooth and commences at the gum. By 15 years of age it reaches half way down the tooth and at 20 it extends the whole length.

Whilst observing the dental stars appearing in place of the cups, the length of Galvayne's groove, and the shape of the tables, one must consider two other important signs. I refer to the length of the teeth and their angle from the jaw.

To summarise, a typical mouth will be as follows:

1 year old: 6 white teeth in lower jaw showing the typical neck of a milk tooth.

2 year old: ditto.

3 year old: 2 central permanent teeth, recognised by their shape, and four milk teeth.

4 year old: 2 central and 2 lateral permanent teeth.

5 year old: 2 central, 2 lateral and 2 corner permanent teeth, the front edges only touching.

6 year old: full mouth with corners in complete opposition, cups visible on all.

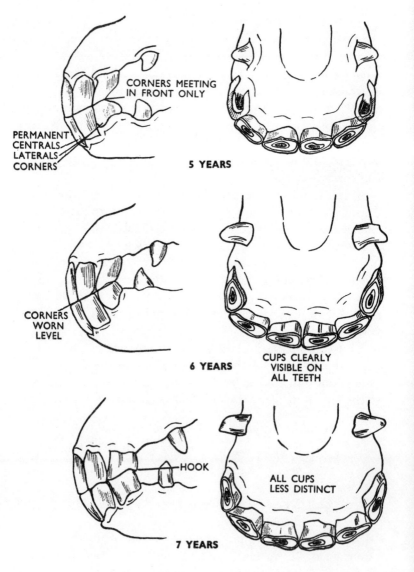

Fig. 9. Teeth

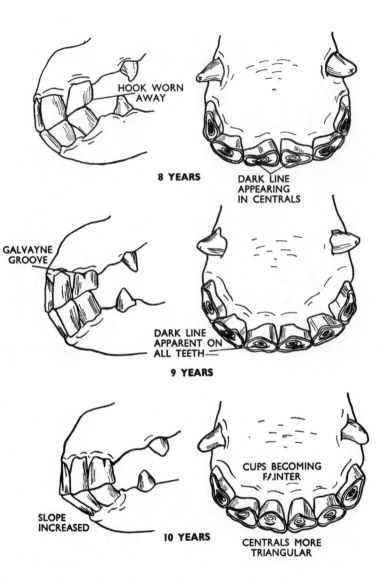

Fig. 10. Teeth

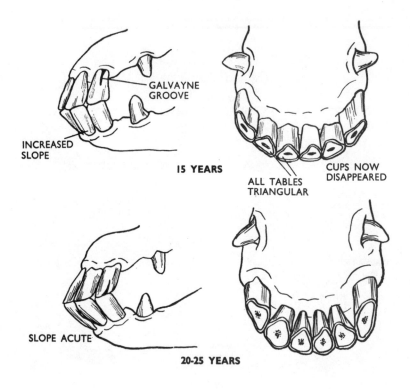

Fig. 11. Teeth

7 year old: full mouth, no cups in centrals, hook on outside
of upper corner incisor.

8 year old: full mouth, no cups on centrals or laterals, but a
small dark area appears in the tables of the
centrals in place of the cups and the hook on the
upper incisor disappears.

9 year old: full mouth, the centrals changing from oval to
triangular. Galvayne's groove on upper corner
incisor, dark spot on the tables of the centrals
and laterals. A nine year old hook on the upper
corner tooth.

10 year old: full mouth, dark spot on all lower incisors, centrals and laterals becoming more triangular, Galvayne's groove about $\frac{1}{4}$ inch long, lower and upper incisors starting to slope forward.

11 year old: full mouth, all incisors assuming triangular shape, Galvayne's groove $\frac{1}{4}$ - $\frac{3}{8}$ of an inch long.

12 year old
13 year old
14 year old
15 year old

Incisors triangular in shape, lower and upper incisors definitely sloping and Galvayne's groove increasing about $\frac{1}{8}$ inch each year.

CHAPTER SIX

General Signs of Health and Disease

Having dealt with the mechanism of the body, I propose to discuss the general signs of health in order that full significance will be given to symptoms of ill-health when discussing disease.

General The animal should be bright and alert with a normal posture and be in fair or good condition. Horses tend to remain standing in daytime but a healthy horse lying down will normally get up when approached.

Coat Except in winter when a horse is turned out to grass, the coat should lie flat and have a certain amount of gloss, or sheen.

Skin The skin should be loose on the underlying tissue and free from excessive scurf.

Eye This should be bright and full. On turning the lids back, the membranes should be a pale salmon pink colour.

Pulse A convenient place to take the rate of the heart beats is on the inner surface of the under jaw. The normal rate should be 35-40 beats per minute in the horse at rest.

Temperature The normal temperature within the rectum is 100°-101.5° F. (37.7-38.6 degrees C).

Urine should be almost colourless.

Droppings The colour and consistency will vary with the diet, but at all times they should be moist and free from any offensive odour.

Limbs should be free from any swelling.

Respiration should be even and regular and at the rate of 8-12 per minute when the horse is at rest. Both the nostrils and the ribs should only move slightly.

Mastication When eating long fodder the grind of the teeth should be even. Examine the food in the manger and if wet, or in 'balls', this is indicative of some defect in the molar or grinding teeth.

Where any variation occurs in the normal signs of health, general indications of disease may be as follows:

General Sick animals appear listless, the head may be lowered with drooping ears, gait and even posture may be unsteady. The horse will be in poor or even in bad condition.

Coat — staring, or on end — general malnutrition, accompanied or otherwise by skin lesions. The coat is the mirror of health of the body.

Examine the mane. In good health the hair is firm in its roots and not easily pulled. Conversely, if one can pull hairs from the mane easily, one should look for other signs of ill health.

Skin — *Tight a.* General malnutrition.

           b. Lice.

           c. The early stages of a general disease.

Sweating. Excessive may be from too much exercise of an unfit animal or from excitement or nervous exhaustion.

Cold sweat. Acute physical pain or mental disturbance.

Hot sweat. Fevers.

Eye — *Pale* membranes denote anaemia from worms or chronic indigestion — internal haemorrhage.

Yellow membranes denote disorders of the liver.

Deep red membranes, known as injected, denote fevers.

Red membranes with a blue tinge are indicative of pneumonia.

Blue red membranes denote heart and circulatory trouble.

Pulse — Increased rate up to 50 per minute may mean pain, but above this rate it usually signifies fever. Irregular beat indicates heart trouble.

Temperature — A rise of 2 or 3 degrees often denotes pain, but above this a general infection should be suspected.

Urine — Thick cloudy urine indicates digestive disturbance or kidney trouble.

Droppings — *Mustard colour.* Liver disorders or Red Worms.

Soft like cow. Indigestion from worms, bad teeth, or bowel infection.

Mucous coated. Irritation of the gut from heated oats or hay, or an infection.

Offensive in smell. Indicates acidity from worms, musty hay, or oats.

Limbs — If generally puffy they may indicate poor circulation from digestive disturbance or heart trouble. If locally puffy there may be a local skin irritation or some underlying bone or joint affliction in which case the animal will go lame.

Respiration — If quicker than 8-12 per minute and laboured may indicate pain, rise in temperature, or pneumonia. Coughing is rare in healthy horses but it may occur due to sore throats, broken wind or even pneumonia.

Mastication — If jerky may denote teeth trouble.

PART II

DISEASE

The subject of disease may now be tackled with some confidence and I am dealing with it under two headings:

1. Non-Specific Diseases: Chapters 7-14.
2. Specific Diseases: Chapter 15.

CHAPTER SEVEN

Inflammation

This has been described by Sanderson as 'the succession of changes occurring in a part as the result of injury insufficient to kill the part'. It is the tissue's reaction to injury or irritation and the clinical signs of inflammation are heat, pain and swelling leading to interference or loss of function.

The first change is an increased flow of blood to the part to bring more food to repair the damaged cells and replace those killed. Very soon, however, as the result of changes in the walls of the veins the circulation slows down. White cells of the blood push their way in large numbers through the capillary walls with large quantities of lymph. The white blood cells attack invading bacteria and remove dead or useless tissues. This increase of blood is evidenced by a swelling. Maybe the artery walls are damaged, causing them to be more porous, and blood oozes out into the part, in which case the swelling is increased. As the exudate forces its way into the tissues it plays an important part in causing pain by simple mechanical stretching actions.

Inflammation is never spontaneous there always being a causal agent, mechanical, chemical or bacterial, but from the patients point of view it is certainly a good thing since the various inflammatory reactions are all directed towards repair. Any treatment adopted should have as its objective the guidance and control of the inflammatory processes rather than any interference with them. The end results of inflammation should be the removal of the irritant by the action of the exudate and the repair of the damaged tissue.

The method of treatment to be adopted in a simple case of inflammation must be directed towards the absorption of dead cells and blood clots (shown in humans by discoloration or bruise). Every effort should be made to keep any bleeding and effusion within limits and at the same time to promote their absorption so as to prevent the collection of stagnant fluids which would delay or complicate recovery. This may be achieved by heat in the form of hot fomentations, which will dilate the blood vessels, bringing more blood for repair by the arteries and increasing the return flow by means of the veins and other vessels.

Heat, however, dilates the veins and lymphatic channels as well. Should this dilation occur to any great extent then the valves present in these vessels may be rendered incompetent and the congestion within the tissues may be increased, especially if there is no muscular movement to aid in the flow.

Cold applications such as hosing with cold water may also be used. These act to stimulate the blood vessels to contract in order to limit the bleeding and fluid exudation and therefore to reduce the swelling and pain. Cold treatment requires to be applied continuously for hours on its own to produce good results.

To relieve pain and congestion therefore, it is common practice to apply alternate warm and cold applications several times during half an hour, causing local dilation and contraction of blood vessels. This produces alternate increase and diminution of the amount of blood passing through the area bringing about an improvement in the physiological efficiency of the tissues.

A further process, the principle of which is applied to many other conditions, is known as osmosis. This is the normal process by which plants feed.

A simple experiment to demonstrate this function is to take any animal tissue, for convenience an animal's bladder, and fill it with a strong solution of sugar or salt, tie the neck to avoid leakage, and immerse it in a weaker solution of salt or sugar in a bucket. It will be seen that the bladder will increase in size and ultimately burst. What happens is that the weak and strong solution pass through the animal tissue, but the weaker solution is attracted to the stronger solution quicker than the reverse.

In applying this to inflamed areas, knowing that the liquid of the body contains about 1 per cent of salts, a stronger solution is applied outside in poultice form – i.e. glycerine and epsom salts, kaolin poultice (salts mixed with a certain mud), etc. This causes attraction of the weaker body fluids through the pores to the stronger solution in the poultice, thereby attracting the inflammatory fluid.

Other possible lines of treatment in inflammatory conditions, particularly of muscles and tendons, includes pressure from correctly applied elastic bandages. These aim at limiting bleeding and effusion with a consequent relief of pain. Hand-rubbing and massage will also relieve pain mechanically and prevent stagnation by aiding the return flow of lymph.

Before leaving the subject of inflammation we should consider the principle of 'blistering', seeing that it is a therapeutic method employed to produce this condition artificially by counter-irritation, i.e. to produce a superficial congestion of the skin and its underlying tissues which may relieve inflammation and congestion in some deeper-seated organ or tissue.

The technique incorporates the use of an irritant to the skin, causing local phenomena; viz. dilation of the arteries, with consequent increase in blood supply to hasten repair of damaged tissue. Veins are dilated and are able to cope with the dead cells and waste products. In the same way the pores being dilated allow of an increase in elimination of waste products.

These phenomena are due directly to the irritant properties of the drug or the direct effect upon the nerves controlling the calibre of the small blood vessels. The friction produced mechanically by the rubbing in of the blister may also have an effect. Resolution of the artificially induced subcutaneous inflammation may attract the original inflammatory exudate and absorb it thereby relieving the deeper-seated inflammation.

The tissue reaction associated with blistering is beneficial in cases of strains. Irritant applications may be employed also for a mechanical effect. It encourages the formation of fibrous tissue, which adds strength to the part.

Bursal enlargements and wind galls may be reduced by the use of a blister, the effect being to thicken the skin. It causes extra tension to be placed on the underlying tissues as would a pressure bandage.

A further use is to assist an indolent abscess to mature and burst. In cases of strangles, the abscess under the jaw is often slow in coming to a head, but the application of a blister will hasten this process.

Blisters are not used so much nowadays for a variety of reasons. The discomfort produced may be such that the horse rests the part as much as possible thus producing congestion since an increased blood flow is produced without necessarily increasing the speed of circulation through the tissues. Since the blister is not usually applied until after the acute stage of an inflammation has passed it may encourage further exudation of fluids. Other and better methods are available such as electrical treatment, in the form of short wave therapy, of which more in a later chapter.

It used to be, and in many places still is, customary to blister a horse's legs after a hard season's hunting or racing in order to 'freshen' them up. Bursal enlargements and minor strains of tendons and ligaments, which develop during the season, are often cured or relieved by a good blistering. The beneficial effect is due to the following:

a. An increased blood supply hastens repair;
b. Pain from the thickened and inflamed skin restricts movement;
c. Tension from the thickened skin acts as a natural bandage.

With regard to the choice of blisters the original red blister has been superseded by a Green non-irritant blister, which is far less severe, and has the great advantage that it is not necessary to tie the animal up for twenty-four hours after application. If a limb is blistered with the non-irritant type the animal may rub it with the cheek and cause a mild inflammation, but this is of no consequence and will subside within a few days.

To summarise, the following points must be observed before applying any blister.

1. Corn and nuts must be discontinued for at least seven days prior to application otherwise a permanent big leg will follow.

2. Where the lower limbs are blistered the hollow of the heels must be liberally greased with vaseline before commencing, otherwise the blister may run on to the delicate skin in the heel and cause severe cracking and considerable pain.

3. Although one leg only needs blistering it is wise to treat both legs, the reason being that, if one leg is treated, the animal will put all its weight on the good leg and might result in strain. If there is any good reason why only one leg is treated it is advisable to apply a stable bandage to the untreated leg to give support to the 'back' tendons.

4. Blistering should not be used in cases of acute inflammation. This should first be reduced by other means, blistering being confined to the sub-acute or chronic inflammatory conditions. Blisters of all kinds should be avoided when a part is in an inflamed or irritable condition.

Firing or the application of the actual cautery to the skin, and in some cases to the deeper tissues as well, is the severest form of counter-irritation, and was often used in the combating of deep-seated chronic inflammatory conditions for which other measures have failed or are thought to be insufficient. Superficial firing produces a similar reaction to blistering although the artificial inflammation produced is much more pronounced. Other types of firing involve more deep-seated action. Owing to the pain and tissue destruction caused by firing, the horse rests the part as much as possible thereby increasing the possibility of congestion. Pressure produced in inflammatory conditions in unyielding tissues like bone may cause serious anaemia which is increased by the loss of muscular action causing a slow up of blood due to resting the part. Firing for the correction of muscle and tendon damage would seem to have little in its favour whereas penetrating point firing of such conditions as ring bone and splints may well be beneficial.

In general both blistering and firing are not used so much nowadays since other and better treatments are available such as short wave therapy.

Finally, the subject of inflammation would not be complete without a general reference to the use of Cortisone. This drug is proving of great value in the treatment of inflammatory conditions of joints, tendons, ligaments, and even bone, and constant reference will be made to its use in such conditions.

There are, however, several grave disadvantages in the use of cortisone, for instance it may delay wound healing and increase the susceptibility to viral infection by suppressing antibody production.

CHAPTER EIGHT

Wounds

A simple wound may be described as a break in the continuity of the skin. Accepting this descriptive explanation, immediately one conjures up a variety of abnormal conditions that will follow. For easy understanding we must consider wounds under several headings.

1. **Simple wounds** of the skin;
2. **Wounds with laceration** and consequent damage to deeper tissues;
3. **Punctured wounds.**

In a simple wound caused by a surgeon's knife, the skin would have been cleansed of all germs and the knife would have been sterilised, thus the healing of such a wound would be an uncomplicated process as follows:

Bleeding would follow from the cut blood vessels which would clot. Lymph containing leucocytes escapes from the blood vessels and coagulates on the wound surface forming a sticky layer which sticks the edges of the wound together. The leucocytes remove dead and damaged tissue. Cells derived from the connective tissue then form at either edge of the wound, and eventually the gap is bridged by this granulation tissue. This new tissue has the power of contracting and in so doing draws the edges together. Skin cells now begin to grow over and cover the wound the whole process being completed in about a week.

A similar process would take place when the object causing the wound was dirty or infected with germs, but the healing would be delayed. The white cells of the blood, which are often called the policemen of the body, would pounce on the invaders and kill or injure those with which they came into contact. The invading germs are not entirely at the mercy of the leucocytes as they can develop powers of resistance and produce a material which clots blood and restricts the flow of lymph, thereby making a protective barrier between themselves and the attacking leucocytes.

Treatment When considering the treatment of wounds it is impossible to lay down fixed methods to suit all occasions. The choice must vary with the type and position of the wound. In the past copious watery dressings and irrigations were used for most wounds, but with the exception of the initial cleansing, this method is no longer used because it hinders healing processes.

The use of strong antiseptics, such as carbolic, iodine, etc., should be discouraged, since they may damage the tissues and interfere with healing. However, the use of certain antiseptics is permissible. Acriflavine is one of the best for wound healing since even in strong solution it is not an irritation to the cells. T.C.P. and Dettol are also useful, but probably the best preparations of all are the Sulphonamides, but care must be taken to use them at the correct strength since below effective strength they may have quite the reverse effect.

The general method of attack should be directed towards assisting the normal reparative functions of the body by:

a. Ensuring a good drainage;
b. Encouraging the flow of blood bringing healing serum to repair damaged tissue and also leucocytes to kill germs;
c. Dealing with infection and preventing further infection;
d. Avoiding damage to the surrounding tissue;
e. Allowing the maximum amount of air compatible with safety.

This technique ensures that the natural healing reactions of the damaged tissue are given every encouragement.

In the case of a simple wound, a primary dressing containing salt, which, by osmosis, will attract the flow of lymph and serum from the cells and stimulate granulation tissue as well as acting as a mechanical cleanser of the area, together with a medicament such as citrate of soda, which will counteract the clotting effect of infection, will be adequate. The proportions are 4 parts of salt to 1 part of citrate of soda, with 1 teaspoonful of this mixture to 1 pint of boiled water. The wound should be cleansed thoroughly of all foreign matter and blood clot. A piece of lint, soaked in the same solution, can be applied to the wound, kept in place by a light bandage and left for twenty-four hours. If an antiseptic dusting powder is available this can be used or an acriflavine solution. It is always advisable to use a layer of cotton wool over the wound so that pressure may be as evenly distributed as possible and so that any bleeding may be checked by coagulation in the meshes of the cotton wool.

On removing the dressing, a yellow sticky mass will be seen covering the wound. This is lymph and should be carefully removed with swabs of cotton wool, soaked in the above solution, and then covered as before.

When washing the wound several small bleeding points will be noticed, which is a good sign. Once the loss of tissue, caused by the wound, is replaced by granulation tissue, i.e. 'proud flesh', a dry dressing should be applied to coagulate the lymph and control the growth of this new tissue. A scab will form, healing will take place under it and the underlying tissue will contract and bring the edges of the wound together.

If the wound is extensive with consequent loss of tissue and deep-seated infection treatment is slightly different. The initial washing of the wound to remove dirt and clotted blood is essential. The next step is to try and remove the infecting germs, which have been implanted in the deeper tissue by the object causing the wound. Penicillin is very effective in such cases and should be applied liberally. A dressing composed of powdered epsom salts, with sufficient glycerine to form a paste, is then smeared on a piece of lint, applied to the wound, covered with oiled silk and bandaged. This dressing should be changed twice daily.

A drawing agent such as the above applied to a deep-seated wound ensures the free flow of serum from the surrounding tissue. This serum has great healing properties and when it is in free flow it is a powerful cleanser of a wound. It is best that an infected wound should heal from within. If healing occurs only in the superficial layers the infection may be imprisoned with unpleasant results.

To ensure the maximum drawing action of a dressing or poultice, the latter must be covered with some waterproof material, such as oiled silk or greaseproof paper, otherwise the poultice will draw its moisture from the air.

If a wound is treated in this way, when the dressing is taken off the tissues will look clean and show several little bleeding points, proving that there is adequate blood supply.

Should the wound be infected with a virulent germ, the patient show systemic disturbance, or the point of entry be so small that a good drainage is not possible, the local treatment must be augmented by injections of penicillin, or other antibiotic, by an expert.

It will be noticed that no reference to stitching has been made, as so often this is not necessary and is not a sound surgical practice. Where a long surface wound has occurred, to avoid excessive scar, stitching is advisable, but as so many wounds in animals are deeply infected, any attempt at stitching before the infection has been drawn out will imprison the latter and is likely to cause a general blood poisoning.

In the event of stitching being resorted to a copious application of penicillin in oil should be applied as deep as possible, and a small portion of the wound left open to ensure drainage.

Most wounds heal more firmly and thoroughly when light exercise is provided. When no exercise is allowed the wound often heals more rapidly but the resulting scar is prone to breakdown or to have restrictive underlying adhesions.

A final word on wound treatment concerns the use of iodine and any of the carbolic antiseptics. These should not be used except in the case of punctured soles, seeing that they coagulate blood and destroy healing tissue. A small packet of sulphanilamide can be carried but most cottages would supply some salt or sugar. Either can be applied to a wound and covered by a stock or bandage until you get home.

SPECIAL WOUNDS

Punctured Wounds affecting a joint or bursa, or likely to spread to the latter, usually from a kick, at the point of the shoulder, just below the elbow, in front of the fetlock, on the stifle, or on the outside of the hock, should be treated by an expert, as once infection reaches any of these joints the animal may be ruined for life.

Punctured wounds of the sole of the foot need special attention. In the first place an injection against lockjaw is essential, as wounds in this region are in contact with material, soil, dung, etc., which often contains tetanus germs, thus making wounds in the foot particularly susceptible to tetanus infection. The next move, and equally essential, is to have the hole caused by the object enlarged to ensure drainage.

No doubt many of us will remember, during our school days, sticking our pen nib into a rubber and noticing that on withdrawing the nib, the hole closed. The same thing happens when hoof tissue is pierced, hence the necessity of cutting down the line of entry until the soft tissue is reached, as evidenced by blood. Most farriers dislike the sight of blood, but you must insist that they go on cutting until the blood is reached.

Having opened and explored the puncture, the foot should be soaked in a bucket of water, to which a handful of salt is added, for about half an hour. The next step is to apply a poultice and a material Col. Codrington found most efficacious is wet brewer's yeast. The sole is packed with this yeast (do not heat) and the foot is wrapped in some mackintosh material, to assist the drawing action, and then covered with a strong sack to prevent damage to the mackintosh. Yeast is not only a powerful drawing agent, but gives off gases, which are lethal to infection. When using brewer's yeast antiseptics should not be used as they will destroy the active fungus of the yeast. The poultice should be changed once or twice daily for at least three days, after which a dry dressing of sulphanilamide may be used. A dry dressing is beneficial at this stage otherwise excessive healing tissue (proud flesh) will be formed in the hole of the sole, and when the latter is closing, it will incorporate and cause pressure on the former resulting in pain and consequent lameness. Stockholm tar may be used in place of sulphanilamide.

You will notice that I have only dealt with punctured wounds in the sole, because in this situation they are generally uncomplicated and a satisfactory recovery may be expected. However, where the foreign object pierces the sensitive frog, the treatment will be the same, but the chances of a complete recovery are less. Providing the foreign object has pierced the horn and the soft tissues covering the pedal bone only, complete recovery may be expected, but if the object has penetrated far enough to damage the pedal bone, recovery may or may not occur. In the same way, should the object have gone deeply into the frog, there is always the chance that the navicular joint has become affected, in which case the animal may be lame permanently.

When the object is embedded in the foot it is necessary, when removing it, to pay particular attention to site and depth of penetration, as this factor will be valuable in assessing the length of time for recovery to take place, if at all. The most dangerous spot is near the point of the frog, for this area is immediately under the coffin joint.

In all deep seated wounds it is a wise and economical practice to give a large dose of one of the long acting antibiotics by injection to block infection gaining access to the system.

Bruises or contusions are injuries to the deeper parts of the skin and subcutaneous tissues. The skin itself is not broken but more or less extensive damage occurs to blood vessels and connective tissue so that blood leaks into the cell spaces of the region. This effusion of blood may produce a swelling with fluid contents. Muscle, tendon and bone may all suffer bruising without any skin wounds. Bone bruising is particularly serious, the blood vessels in the periosteum covering the bone surface being damaged. The reparative processes give rise to new bone tissue (exostoses) which may subsequently interfere with free movement. With reference to bone a small surface contusion may actually mask a fracture of the underlying bone, this will be mentioned later.

Over-Reach This is caused by the hind shoe lacerating:
(*a*) the bulbs of the heel, and
(*b*) the back of the fetlock joint.

(*a*) Where the bulb of the heel is concerned. owing to the tissues in this area being poorly supplied with blood, healing is slow.

Treatment Often there is a flap of skin and tissue torn almost completely away. and this should be removed, as there is small chance of union taking place. If left it will form a blemish.

Then the wound should be cleansed thoroughly with salt and water, and a poultice of brewer's yeast applied daily, as in the case of a punctured sole, for a week. To avoid excessive formation of healing tissue, once it has filled the gap formed by the loss, dry dressings should be resorted to, such as sulphanilamide. If excessive healing tissue is formed a little powdered blue stone, dusted on daily, will arrest further formation.

(*b*) where the over-reach affects the fetlock, or lower third of the tendons, generally this is much more serious.

If one considers the position of the fore leg at the time of an over-reach, fixed on the ground and the tendon taut, the extensive damage to the latter, which invariably occurs, will be understood. Often this skin wound is misleading in that it is comparatively small and bears no relation to the extent of the damage.

In all cases where there is a fair sized wound in the skin (about 1 inch long), it is almost certain that the sheath of the tendon is either broken or so extensively damaged that it will burst. If this has happened copious discharge of a yellow sticky fluid will be seen on the edges of the wound. This fluid is from the tendon sheath and it is called synovia. It is similar to 'joint oil' in function and character.

Treatment To avoid blemish, one may be tempted to stitch these wounds, but I consider that it is unwise to do so. The aim must be to allow infecting germs, extraneous material and dead cells to escape from the deeper tissues, in order to avoid further infection to the tendon and its sheath.

Once the wound has been cleansed thoroughly with salt water, brewer's yeast should be applied *and a Veterinary Surgeon called.*

Punctured Wounds on the inside of the second thigh, a favourite place for kicks, need a special note, if only as a warning.

The bone is covered only by the skin and a little connective tissue in this area and in consequence it is extremely vulnerable to injury. The wound may appear small and heal fairly quickly and the horse may show no lameness, yet often there is extensive damage to the bone. The outer casing may be splintered in the form of a star, the cracks radiating out from the point of contact. As the animal is sound it may be sent out for exercise, or in the case of a horse at grass, turned out again. Because this splintering of the casing has weakened the bone, fast work may result in a complete fracture.

Warning – where wounds occur in this position, whether the animal is lame or not, it is best to presume that the bone may be seriously injured. The horse should be kept at rest for at least twenty-one days to ensure healing of the bone.

Broken Knees This is the term used to describe any injury to the front of the knees, generally occasioned from falling.

The extent of the damage to the skin and underlying tissue is the governing factor in making a prognosis.

A slight graze, whereby the hair is removed, may recover without any visible defect, but if the damage to tissues is deep seated and the hair follicles destroyed a permanent scar will result. This in itself may not interfere with action at all, but in a show horse or to a prospective buyer it might suggest that the animal is liable to stumble — a most unpleasant defect. *Ask your Veterinary Surgeon to examine the heart as it may be the primary cause of the trouble.*

Treatment This varies according to the extent of the injury.

If the graze has not penetrated the skin, but merely removed the surface hair, bathing the wounds with cold salt water for a week will effect a cure.

Where the skin has been broken, as evidenced by blood and a yellow liquid discharge, usually some gravel or dirt has been forced into the tissues. This should be drawn out with a poultice. A paste made of glycerine and epsom salts, smeared on a piece of lint about one-eighth of an inch thick, should be applied to the wound and kept in place by a light bandage. This dressing should be applied twice a day for three days, after which an antiseptic ointment should be applied and the wound allowed to scab. If the hair does not appear to be growing it may be worth while to try the effect of a stimulant application, containing cantharides.

Should the damage be extensive and the ligaments, or even the bone, be exposed the treatment must be more vigorous. At the outset a poultice of glycerine and epsom salts should be applied for the first three days to draw out any gravel in the tissues. Hose with cold water twenty minutes two or three times a day for a week to reduce the inflammation, after which the part can be dressed with an antiseptic oil dressing, such as acriflavine emulsion, applied twice daily. It may be necessary for the animal to be tied up, or even put in slings, to prevent it from lying down and so breaking the healing tissue.

After the wound has healed sufficiently exercise is indicated in order to prevent adhesions between the surfaces of the joint membranes should these have been damaged. Adhesions will consequently limit the movement of the joint. No joint should be kept immobilised for an indefinite or prolonged period.

Whatever the extent of the injury or the treatment, remember two things. Do not use hot applications to a knee, or hock, and do not apply bandages to keep any dressings in position for more than three days, as either will increase the inflammation and especially the latter. Even if an adequate 'buffer' of cotton wool be used, the prominent bone at the back of the knee will soon become inflamed and cause as much trouble as the wound itself.

Thorn Injuries As a routine measure when a horse returns from hunting or chasing, once the mud has been roughly removed with straw, a careful search should be made for thorns. Sometimes they can be found and removed easily, but the tendency is for them to break off at the level of the skin if care is not taken, especially in the case of black thorns. If a thorn is located the hair should be cut around the point of entry and, if it cannot be withdrawn, it should be cut out by an expert at once. So often a poultice is applied with no result, the sequel being a big leg for some time.

Since the advent of penicillin and streptomycin often an infection due to a thorn can be cleared up in no time by a course of injections of same, without the long and tedious hot fomentations used in the past, but this fact should not deter every effort being made to remove the thorn at the time. Once the thorn has been removed a poultice should be applied at once to draw out the infection that will have been implanted in the deeper tissues.

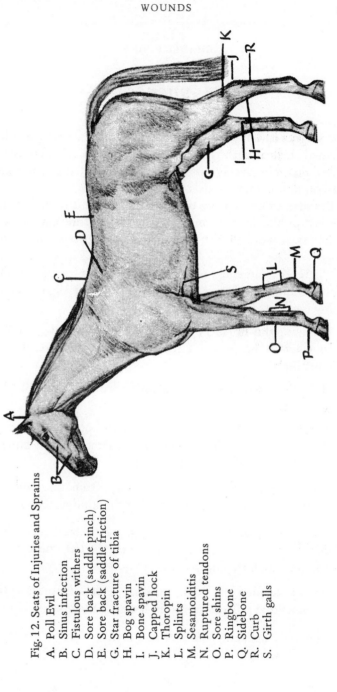

Fig. 12. Seats of Injuries and Sprains
A. Poll Evil
B. Sinus infection
C. Fistulous withers
D. Sore back (saddle pinch)
E. Sore back (saddle friction)
G. Star fracture of tibia
H. Bog spavin
I. Bone spavin
J. Capped hock
K. Thoropin
L. Splints
M. Sesamoiditis
N. Ruptured tendons
O. Sore shins
P. Ringbone
Q. Sidebone
R. Curb
S. Girth galls

CHAPTER NINE

Lameness

The subject of lameness is so vast and complicated that I have decided to deal with the common types and causes only, and where possible give symptoms that are peculiar to the area to aid you in locating the part affected.

Because there appears to be considerable difficulty among the lay public in differentiating between fore and hind leg lameness, a word or two on general principles should not be amiss.

Where the lameness is acute the selection of the unsound limb should be obvious, but often it is so slight that the following hints to diagnosis may be of value.

a. Examine the horse in his stall paying particular attention to whether he points a forelimb, if so this would be the lame limb.

b. Have the horse trotted up, stand in front of the animal and concentrate on the fore legs.

c. Watch the head and if the level of the poll appears to rise and fall one of the fore limbs is affected, the lame leg being the one on which the poll rises.

d. Now have the horse trotted away from you and concentrate on the 'jumping bump' in the hind quarters.

e. If the level of this 'bump' appears to rise and fall the lameness is in the hind limbs, the affected one being the one on which the hip rises.

Having decided the limb, there are certain features as to its movement that will assist you in locating the area.

Generally speaking the gait and stance peculiar to an area are as follows:

Shoulder When moving, the affected limb is not extended as far forward as the sound limb, the toe is dragged and the neck muscles come into play more prominently to assist the forward movement of the limb. When at rest the affected limb is often held behind the sound one with the toe resting on the ground.

Elbow In movement the weight is taken first on the toe with the knee slightly bent. When standing the elbow is dropped and the knee and fetlock bent.

Cannon Splint — The affected limb appears to be carried further away from the body than its fellow.
Sore Shins — A very short step and a swinging of the limb when brought forward. Stance is inclined to be over at the knee.

Pastern Ringbone — a short stilty step. On moving sideways or turning lameness is accentuated.

Foot Corn — very similar to splint lameness.
Navicular Disease — short 'punchy' strides.

Hip A short step on the toe, exaggerated lift of the haunch.

Stifle Again a shorter step on the toe, with rotation of the joint outward. If the pace is quickened the limb will often be carried. When at rest the limb is often lifted and from time to time carried with the stifle flexed.

Hock An exaggerated raising of the hips by the sound leg and dragging of the toe of the affected leg.

It must be clearly understood that the above hints regarding location are very rough and are offered as a general guide. Details and peculiarities of lameness will be dealt with separately below.

Shoulder A diagnosis of shoulder lameness has often been the subject of some derision, it being said that when the cause of lameness is obscure, the shoulder is suggested as a last resort.

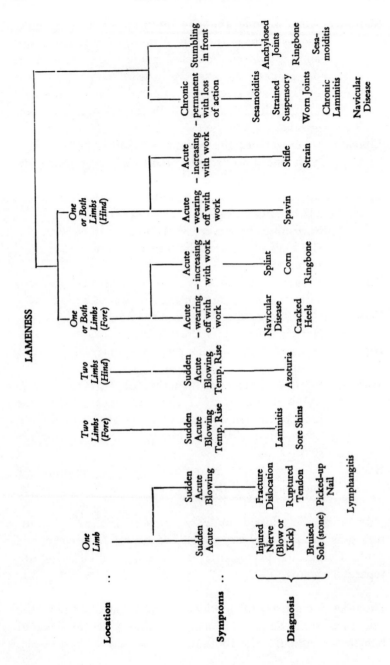

For every case of geniune lameness in the shoulder there are at least fifty in other parts of the limb, but this does not alter the fact that shoulder lameness does occur.

Quite often the joint is jarred when jumping dropped fences, and in the case of flat race horses, working too much on one track. The only other general cause is bruising of the point by a kick or running into an object.

Diagnosis Except where a definite swelling is present on the point of the shoulder due to injury, an exact diagnosis is too difficult for the layman and in consequence it and *treatment must be left to a Veterinary Surgeon.* The value of Short Wave Therapy will be dealt with under a separate heading.

Elbow Similar remarks apply to this area as to the shoulder.

Cannon — Splint Besides the main cannon bone, there are two small vestigial bones at the back of it known as splint bones. At birth these bones are quite separate, but at varying times up to four years old they unite with the main bone.

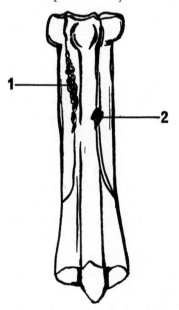

Fig. 13.
Cannon bone showing several splints (1) running into each other and a single (2) splint. Splints are found in the forelimbs more commonly and on the inside more often than the outside of the limb.

Before unity takes place there is movement between these bones. If excessive work is given, especially on hard ground, the normal process of bony growth forming to unite the bones is exaggerated and this outgrowth is known as a splint.

It has just been suggested that excessive concussion before the horse is mature may be the prime contributory factor to the incidence of the condition. Other factors may play a part, such as brushing or cutting and therefore striking the cannon with the shoe of the other foot. Defects of conformation such as knock-knees or bandy-legs will throw extra strain on the inside or the outside of the limb and cannon in particular, and therefore on the corresponding small splint bones. Faulty shoeing may well throw similar strains on the inside or the outside of the knee. Finally there may be an hereditary predisposition.

Diagnosis In considering splint lameness one must remember that only occasionally does it occur in a horse over five years old. The limb appears to be carried away from the body, lameness is aggravated on rough ground, and often it develops with work. Lameness normally appears before any bony enlargement can be seen or felt, although pressure in the region will produce pain.

On lifting the leg, with the knee fully flexed, it is generally possible to feel a splint, by running one's thumb down between the edge of the suspensory ligament and the splint bone. If a splint is forming it will be felt as a spongy swelling with some heat and the animal evinces considerable pain on *slight* pressure. However, it must be realised that splints often form without lameness, and when examining the leg these may be felt, but are quite cold and hard and should not be confused with an active splint causing lameness. Remember one can often make an animal flinch if considerable pressure is applied with the thumb, as the main nerve runs down the cannon in this area and may be pinched.

Treatment If the patient is rested the inflammatory process will abate, but on resumption of work the lameness will recur, thus rest is not indicated. Providing the lameness is not acute walking exercise is preferable to hasten the process to finality. If lameness persists an injection of one of the Cortisone preparations in and around the actual swelling will quickly reduce the inflammation and hasten the hardening off. A further injection may be necessary after five days. However, cortisone injections will not correct the cause and the periostitis may well become more severe after the injections have ceased. The application of a mild blister, or even firing, is employed to harden off the process but both have the disadvantage that, over-stimulation of the inflammation can result in an excessive growth of bone, which sometimes presses on the main nerve and accentuates the lameness, or could be unsightly.

Sore Shins This is an inflammatory condition of the membrane or periosteum of the cannon bones, usually in the forelimbs, and marked by swelling and great tenderness. Viewed from the side the cannon bone appears to be 'bowed'. Usually it is seen in two to three-year-old thoroughbred horses and is supposed to be due to the effect of concussion upon immature bone. Curiously it is observed also in young arab horses that work on soft ground only.

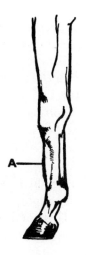

Fig. 14. Sore shins showing the painful diffuse swelling (A) at the front of the cannon bone.

There is no difficulty in diagnosis as the swelling is perceptible and the pain is obvious, even when passing the fingers lightly down the bone.

Treatment The animal should be rested, given a laxative, and all corn stopped.

To allay the inflammation antiphlogistine, or kaolin poultice, should be applied for a week. This may be followed by a mild blister. When the condition is slight, gentle massage with iodine ointment or painting daily with 5 per cent iodine in glycerine may suffice.

The trouble varies in degree, but in all cases the animal should not be worked for at least a month.

Sesamoiditis In the formation of the fetlock joint, besides the cannon and first pastern bone, there are two bones which articulate on the lower end of the cannon and are known as sesamoid bones. They act as a fulcrum to the back tendons since these tendons pass over their hind surfaces within a sesamoid synovial sheath on their way down to the pedal bone. The suspensory ligament is attached to both sesamoids and they in turn are attached by numerous ligaments to the lower end of the cannon bone and to the long pastern bone. This whole area is therefore extremely complicated and liable to damage.

Through concussion and over-extension of the joint these bones may be injured and become inflamed. The covering membrane or skin of the bone throws out new bone, which may incorporate and interfere with the ligaments. The various sesamoidean ligaments may also themselves be strained or even torn away from the bone resulting in a periostitis. There is a tendency for the condition to become chronic.

Symptoms Pain, swelling and lameness. On examination of the back and sides of the fetlock joint it will be found to be enlarged, the swelling being hard as compared with a strained joint when the swelling is soft. This condition seldom occurs suddenly but is slow in onset and progressive.

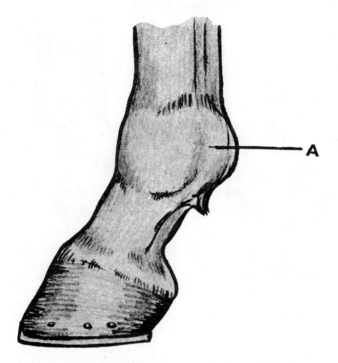

Fig. 15. A. Sesamoiditis. Showing the position of the hard swelling at the back-and sides of the fetlock joint.

Treatment If the lameness is acute the joint must be immobilized with a tight support bandage. Corrective shoeing elevating the heels may relieve the tension on the sesamoids but it will recur when normal shoes are reapplied. Rest and a good blistering may effect a cure, but often the condition recurs with work and the animal develops a short pottery action.

Pastern — Ringbone This is a condition affecting the bones of the pastern — viz. the two bones which run from the fetlock joint to the pedal bone. The covering membrane of either bone may be injured and become inflamed, due to concussion, and a bony outgrowth follows. If this outgrowth

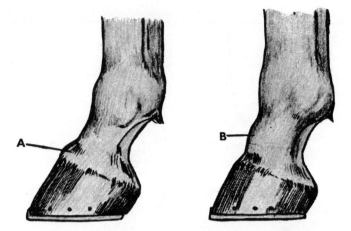

Fig. 16. Ringbone. A. Low ringbone occurring around the coffin joint. At first there is no outward palpable or visible sign; after a time the hoof bulges at the coronet where the deposit of bone pushes the coronet, and wall which grows from it, outwards. B. High ringbone occurring around the pastern joint. The exostosis can usually be seen and felt from the onset of the condition.

affects the part where a tendon moves over the bone, or if it involves a joint, lameness will occur. It is more common in the forefeet owing to the greater stresses imposed on these during movement and occurs more often in heavier or aged horses being rare in less than a four year old.

Diagnosis If excessive the growth may be felt and there will be heat in the area. A typical lameness is seen when the animal is walked on rough ground, if turned short, or moved from side to side.

Treatment If the condition is caused by an injury, rest and ordinary treatment for the inflammation may effect a cure.

Corticosteroid may be injected into joints to relieve pain but its effects are only temporary and of limited value. Once new growths of bone have formed it is impossible to remove them so that an absolute cure is never possible.

If the condition occurs as a result of concussion from work, rest and blistering may arrest the inflammatory process, although blistering in the early stages of the condition may have the opposite effect and promote even greater amounts of bone formation. Electrical treatment has also effected many cures. However, if the process involves the ligaments of the joint, or the joint itself, the prospects of recovery are poor.

The joint affected almost always ends by becoming stiff due to fusion between the bones the joint being obliterated. Any pain occasioned by movement of the joint will therefore disappear and the horse may become fairly sound although it will always have a stiff and stilted gait. This joint fusion can be accelerated by confining the horse for a prolonged period in its stall or even by using a plaster cast.

Laminitis To appreciate this condition one must first consider the structure of the foot. On the inner surface of the wall of the horn are numerous leaves, or laminae, which interlock with corresponding laminae covering the front of the pedal bone. This inter-locking holds the pedal bone in position more or less suspended above the frog. These leaves have a large blood supply and in consequence, should anything occur to suddenly increase the flow of blood to the foot, congestion occurs, as, unlike soft tissues, the hoof is unable to expand. The laminae become swollen and forced apart, especially at the toe, but those at the heel often remain interlocked. The toe of the pedal bone, having lost its attachments, drops, presses on the sole and causes the latter to become flat or even convex. The condition can affect all four feet.

The direct causes are concussion from fast work on hard ground. The indirect causes are constitutional or metabolic and are often associated with disturbances from excessive concentrated foods, standing about in very cold weather when sweating, and the ingestion of a large amount of cold water when very hot. Insufficient exercise, overweight, idleness for long periods will all be predisposing causes.

The condition is also prevalent among small ponies running on very good pasture. These ponies so often get over fat and

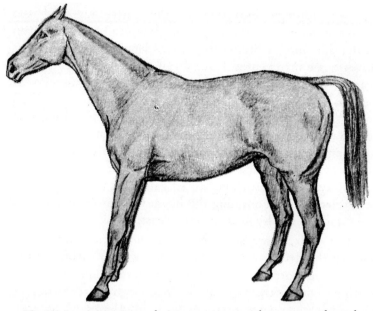

Fig. 17. Laminitis: General picture to suggest the posture adopted. The hind legs are well forward to take the weight off the fore legs and the fore legs are extended throwing the weight on the heels. The horse is rooted to the spot with an agonized facial expression, widely dilated pupils, injected membranes and trumpet shaped nostrils. The body trembles with pain and sweats profusely, respiration is distressed and the pulse increases.

this, together with lack of constant attention to the feet, will invariably result in an attack.

Symptoms One must consider an acute and chronic type in discussing symptoms.

Acute This form occurs quite suddenly and the animal appears to be rooted to the spot. If the fore legs only are affected the animal gets its hind feet as far underneath him as possible to relieve the weight on the fore feet. This stance might lead to confusion, the owner thinking that the animal was suffering from some injury to the back. If made to turn, he will use his hind legs in such a way that he appears to be lifting his forehand round, the fore feet touching the ground lightly at the heel only.

On account of the fact that normally the sensitive foot is such a perfect fit inside the horny box, the latter will not yield to accommodate the extra blood, hence the acute pain evidenced in this disease. Other signs of pain are usually present, such as blowing, sweating, and a rise in temperature.

Chronic Because a chronic case is often the outcome of an acute attack, movement is similar, but it does not occasion so much pain. The back muscles come into action to relieve weight on the forehand and the animal walks on his heel. Due to this, a slow progressive change may occur in the shape of the foot. The toe elongates and the heels and pasterns become vertical. The pedal bone tip presses on the horn of the sole behind the toe and in extreme cases may penetrate through.

Treatment *Because the cause of this disease is often a complicated circulatory failure, a Veterinary Surgeon must be called in at once.* Appropriate treatment in the very early stages may effect a complete cure in a very short time.

As a first-aid measure to the horse in great pain ice cold poultices applied to the feet will relieve congestion to a certain extent and reduce the pain.

As stated earlier, small moorland and shetland ponies are susceptible subjects, especially when grazing on rich pasture and given little work. Failure to have the feet cut down well at least once a month to allow maximum frog pressure predisposes to the condition also. If these points are watched, many cases will be prevented.

If a case does develop, even to the extent that the pony cannot move, Col. Codrington suggested that many cases will recover if the following routine is carried out. The pony must be moved from the rich pasture to a yard or poor keep, if necessary by box. The feet must be cut down drastically and the pony forcibly walked on hard ground or road until the action commences to return, usually after seven to ten days. This might appear cruel but I do not consider it is if the outcome is a cure, seeing that it is the only method of relieving congestion in the feet and restoring normal circulation. When walking freely the pony may be shod but work must be maintained and constant attention given to the feet. If the pasture is comparatively rich grazing must be restricted to one to two hours daily.

Navicular Disease In the formation of the pedal joint, besides the articulation between the short pastern bone and the pedal bone, there is a small shuttle-shaped bone lying against the back of the short pastern bone. Its use is to act as a fulcrum for the deep tendon before it joins the under surface of the pedal bone. At either end of the bone is a ligament joining it to the wings of the pedal bone. This bone may become diseased, principally on the surface over which the deep tendon passes. The area becomes pitted and roughened.

The direct causes of navicular disease are still not known but it may be due to an hereditary predisposition, together with concussion and injury arising from work. Many contributory causes have been suggested, such as lack of frog pressure, bad shoeing, whereby the heels are allowed to contract, and toe growth so allowing undue strain to be thrown on the back tendons. It has also been suggested that toxic absorption during or after influenza or strangles may act as a causative agent by altering the bone density and rendering it less liable to withstand stress.

Diagnosis Because symptoms of this disease vary so much between the initial stages and the advanced case, diagnosis must be considered in each stage.

Thanks to X-ray a more definite diagnosis may be made at an early stage. Small roughened or pitted areas may be seen on the bone, but even before this has occurred, it is often possible to see that the ligaments at the ends of the bone are becoming ossified. When this occurs the bone is less resilient and consequently the concussion is greater. Col. Codrington noticed this on a number of occasions where he X-rayed cases of foot lameness showing no recognised clinical symptom.

Generally the history of these cases is a foot lameness with no apparent cause and it is temporary. After a varying time the animal goes sound and may remain so for several months, but eventually the lameness returns, definite diseased areas of the bone are seen on X-ray, and typical symptoms occur. Both feet are often affected and the animal goes on his heels, taking a shorter stride than normal. At rest one, or both limbs, as the case may be, are extended alternately to relieve the tension of the tendon on the bone, known as 'pointing'. On moving, the lameness is acute at first, but is less as the animal warms up. If allowed to stand for a while after exercise acute lameness returns. If the shoe is examined it is

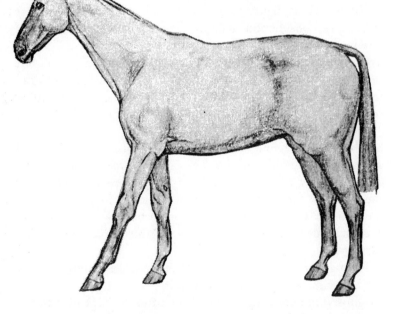

Fig. 18. Navicular disease: 'Pointing' the first marked symptom of navicular disease consists of the horse resting the affected foot (or feet) by placing it a short distance in front of the other when standing in the stable. When both feet are affected the horse points each in turn.

seen to be more worn at the toe than at the heels. When turning around the horse pivots on the forefeet so that he won't have to raise them from the ground.

Treatment Unfortunately there is no cure for this disease. Shoeing with leather to minimise concussion may be adopted, but only as a palliative.

Pedal Ostitis As its name implies this is an inflammatory condition of the pedal bone caused by jar or excessive work on hard ground. It may be the sequel to corns, laminitis or punctures of the sole.

The symptoms are similar to an early case of Navicular Disease in the type of lameness but differs in that it is acute and occurs suddenly, is aggravated by exercise, there is heat in the foot, and slight tapping of the sole with a light hammer will cause considerable pain, and finally it is usual to affect one foot only.

Treatment Rest and poulticing have shown good results but the injection of one or two doses of Cortisone deep into the foot at the hollow of the heel will often show good and quick results. Advanced cases are, however, basically incurable.

Sidebones The name sidebone has been given to an ossified cartilage at the side of the foot. These cartilages arise from either wing of the pedal bone and act as a shock-absorber for the sensitive foot. Concussion first causes an inflammation at their union to the wings of the pedal bone and ossification occurs, which eventually spreads to the remainder of the cartilage.

Riding horses do not often suffer from this condition, but the heavy hunter type is subject to it.

Diagnosis Lameness does not occur often, except possibly in the initial stages.

On examining the bulbs of the heel and the area immediately above the hoof in front of them, the cartilages may be felt and will yield to pressure if they are normal. If ossification has taken place, flexion and resilience will be

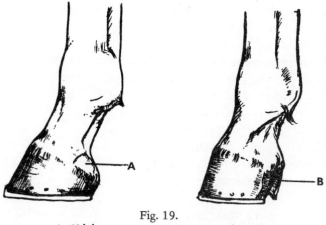

Fig. 19.

A. Sidebone   B. Contracted Heel

impeded and the hard bony deposit may be felt.

Treatment As lameness is negligible no treatment is necessary. If the foot is normal otherwise, sidebones rarely cause lameness.

Contracted Heels This is the name of a condition which is shown by narrowing of the heels or even the entire foot and normally occurring at the front. It results from the drying out of the horny wall by excessive rasping of its outer surface or from lack of frog pressure due to neglect of foot care or as a sequel to a chronic case of thrush in which the entire frog is involved.

Treatment The object is to re-establish normal frog pressure. The horny wall at the heels and quarters is cut back to the normal level and some type of special shoe may be fitted, tips for instance allow maximum frog pressure, or shoeing with a rubber frog pad or even a frog bar.

Thrush This is a condition in which the glands of the sensitive frog 'sweat' excessively, due to irritation from dirt, stale urine, etc. Usually it is seen in the hind feet, but the fore feet may be affected. The cleft of the frog is moist and a characteristic foetid smell is always present.

Treatment The cleft of the frog should be opened up and a dressing of stockholm tar, copper sulphate, alum, or other astringent powders applied.

The main reason for the condition resisting treatment is that the dressings are not applied deeply. After the dressing has been applied a piece of string drawn backwards and forwards will ensure the medicament reaching the affected parts.

Preventive measures should be directed towards stable cleanliness and frequent attention to the feet — washing with disinfectant and paring.

Corns A corn is a name given to a bruise of the sensitive foot, due to pressure. The site is at an angle formed by the wall of the hoof and the bar. Generally it is seen in the fore feet only and mostly on the inside. The pressure causing corns may come from the shoes, the horn of the sole overgrowing so much that is presses upon the shoe, or possibly stones may become wedged between the heel of the shoe and the seat of corn. The pressure causes bruising of the deeper sensitive tissues and the blood vessels become more porous and may even rupture, allowing the blood to exude and permeate into the deeper layers of the horn. Some horses appear to be more susceptible to corns than others.

Symptoms Varying degrees of lameness, which becomes acute on uneven ground, heat around the heels, and on moving, the affected limb appears to be carried away from the body. Tapping the area with a hammer may cause flinching. When made to walk the horse does so by using the toe of the affected foot keeping the heel raised from the ground.

Diagnosis Removal of the shoe and cutting the horn to reveal the bruise is the direct method.

Treatment All bruised sole should be removed if possible and a poultice applied for four to five days to draw away any inflammatory fluid. A *seated shoe* should be fitted to avoid further pressure and the blacksmith warned to search for corns at subsequent shoeings. A three-quarter shoe is favoured by some, but this affords no protection against treading on stones, etc.

When the corn has been neglected the part may become infected, and often there is a minute channel running up into the sensitive structures – 'a piping corn'. In this case the 'pipe' must be followed up and cut out, the foot soaked once or twice daily in a bucket of cold disinfectant water before poulticing, and this treatment continued for a longer period.

If the horse has not been immunized against tetanus this should be done without delay.

Seedy Toe This condition is one in which the wall of the foot separates from the sole at the toe, the space formed being filled with a soft crumbling horn. The cause is often difficult to assign, although pressure of some kind such as a tightly hammered back toe-clip or a tightly driven nail appear to be the most likely.

The condition may not be noticed until the time of shoeing because in the early stages no lameness occurs, but once observed all the cheesy horn must be cut away before recovery can take place. If the cavity is not deep this may be done from the sole, but where the case has been neglected the depth of the cavity is such that the wall must be removed to allow all the dead horn to be cut away.

In any case, once the cheesy bone has been removed the cavity should be packed with an antispetic paste, such as B.I.P. This consists of Bismuth Carbonate – 3 parts, Iodoform – 1 part, made into a thick paste with liquid paraffin. The hole should then be plugged with tow and where possible the shoe put on again.

An application of Cornucrescine to the coronet is beneficial, as it will increase the growth of horn.

Canker Owing to advancement of stable hygiene this conditions is rarely seen these days. Another reason for its rarity is that canker is a chronic disease and often incurable and it

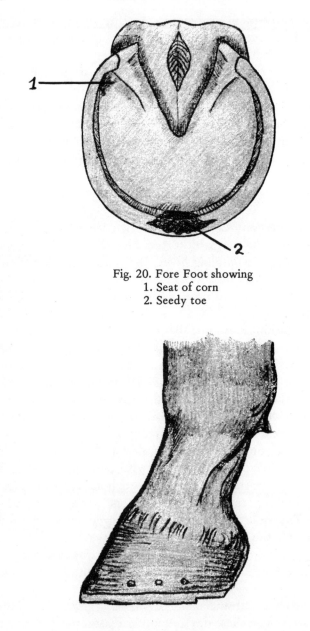

Fig. 20. Fore Foot showing
1. Seat of corn
2. Seedy toe

Fig. 21. Cut Away Shoe for Corn

does interfere with the efficiency of the horse. Most modern owners cannot be bothered with horses which are liable to spend long periods away from work and they therefore cut their losses and destroy them.

Canker is basically an affliction of the horn secreting tissues so that any horn subsequently produced is of a soft cheesy nature. If the hoof is continuously kept damp it may soften and swell and undergo some degree of decomposition so that varieties of germs gain entrance below the horn and set up irritation and subsequent slow inflammation producing the abnormal, soft horn growth.

Cause From standing in dirty ill-drained stables with the hind feet in contact with stale urine and litter soiled with droppings. Support for this theory is the fact that the condition is most common in the hind feet. Rarely is it found in light horses.

Symptoms The sole is moist and areas of horn are under run. There is a characteristic foetid odour. In an advanced case areas of horn are absent and the underlying sensitive sole can be seen.

Treatment This is speculative and in most cases economically unsound. All diseased tissue should be removed and the foot bandaged in an antiseptic pack. Aureomycin powder applied to the sole directly followed by bandaging may have beneficial effects but the bandaging must be continuously applied until the wound heals which may be months.

Sandcrack For some unknown reason a split in the wall of the foot is known as a sandcrack. It may occur in any foot and extends from the coronet downwards. Anything which actually interferes with the proper nutrition of the horn at the coronet may be the cause of it. Lameness may or may not be associated with it, depending on the depth and extent of the crack. If the sensitive tissues are involved inflammation may ensue or the sensitive structures may be pinched between the two edges of the crack. In either case the horse will be lame and characterised by a sudden jerk when the horse raises the foot from the ground.

Treatment Where the crack does not extend the whole length of the wall a V-shaped groove made at the base of the crack will immobilise the portions of horn and facilitate healing. A clip may be used for the same purpose. Should the crack reach to the bottom of the wall a useful method of immobilising the parts is to ease the wall of the foot below the crack so that one can pass a worn penny between that part of the hoof and the shoe.

A useful addition to the above mechanical treatment is the application of a stimulant to increase the growth of horn. Equal parts of cod liver oil, whale oil, Neat's Foot Oil, and castor oil massaged into the coronet, wall, and sole daily for several weeks will have a very beneficial effect.

Stifle Slip Actual lameness in the stifle joint has been dealt with but the condition under discussion here is a dislocation. On the front of the stifle is the patella which corresponds to our knee cap. This bone is held in position by several ligaments and moves in a groove on the bottom of the femur. Due to a sudden false step, becoming tangled up in wire, etc., the patella slips out of the groove. The stifle is held in a semiflexed position and the animal refuses to put any weight on it. Sometimes the bone can be felt on the outside of the joint.

Another condition occurs in the stifle joints of many horses as a normal occurrence. The patella is hooked upwards and over the medial lip of the femoral trochlea and the stifle is locked in position as part of the 'stay apparatus' whereby the animal can remain standing using a reduced level of muscular effort. This is not a true luxation but can occur in young horses before the bones have attained their adult size relationships and will produce involuntary locking of the leg in an extended position.

Treatment If a Veterinary Surgeon is not available the bone can be put back occasionally in the following way.

One end of a piece of rope is tied round the horse's neck. The other end is passed round the heel and back up through

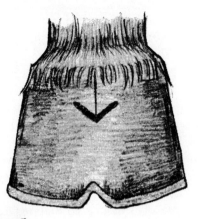

Fig. 22. Sandcrack, showing V-shaped groove cut in wall at the base of the crack.

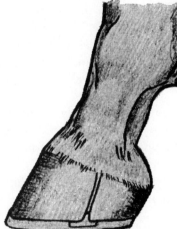

Fig. 23. Sandcrack appearing on the side of the wall. The shoe is seated to isolate the break.

the loop on the neck. When the rope is pulled the leg is pulled forwards and upwards. The animal will resist but if a steady pull is maintained the toe can be brought almost to the level of the elbow when the patella will usually slip back into the groove.

After the dislocation has been reduced short bedding should be used as movement of the limb will be restricted through pain and in consequence long straw may become wound round the foot and cause a recurrence. According to the length of time the bone is dislocated a variable amount of inflammatory swelling will occur and this can be treated by hot fomentations for two to three days followed by the application of a stimulant liniment.

Dislocation of the patella may occur in yearlings and two-year-olds without any previous false step or injury. Usually the type of colt that is affected is one that has been fed well, and grown rather quickly, especially those that have been kept in the stable preparatory to a show or sale.

The animal is usually found rooted to the spot and no amount of persuasion will move him. There are no general symptoms such as blowing, sweating or temperature.

The best method of dealing with these cases, especially if the box is small, is to manoeuvre the patient until its head is facing the door, put plenty of bedding in the doorway and outside the box, and crack a whip or give it a slap on the quarters with a flat stick. Usually the animal will jump and you may actually hear the report of the patella going back into position. Invariably the patient will walk away quite sound.

Once this condition has occurred it is likely to happen again especially if the colt is not given plenty of exercise. Where possible the colt should be turned out. Fortunately the condition is one that most colts will outgrow.

Spavin is the name given to a bony enlargement on the inside of the hock resulting from inflammation of one or more bones in this area.

The inflammation affects the head of the inner splint bone first and spreads upwards to the bones of the hock in the immediate vicinity. The final result is fusion of the affected bones.

The cause of the condition is still controversial but there certainly appears to be an hereditary predisposition to spavin. Apart from this, inflammation of some of the soft structures in the hock region may spread to the periosteum of the bone, or excessive concussion due to overwork, hard surfaces, faulty shoeing or the like, may induce it.

Conformation of the joint appears to have little effect on the incidence of the condition.

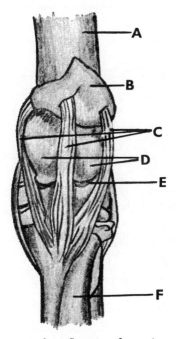

Fig. 24. Left Stifle Joint, front view

A. Femur
B. Patella
C. Ligaments holding patella
   in D
D. Rounded articular surfaces on end
   of femur in which patella moves
E. Joint between femur and
F. Tibia

Confusion in diagnosis may occur where the heads of the splint bones are unduly large, but as spavin occurs in one limb at a time usually, comparison of both hocks should help. In a normal hock a groove, running obliquely downwards and inwards, may be felt over the spavin area and if this is not present, due to its being filled up with inflammatory bone tissue, a spavin may be suspected.

Symptoms Lameness occurs when the animal moves off after standing and diminishes with exercise. If the case is recent lameness may be evident only when the horse is first moved after resting from fast work.

Flexion of the hock causes pain and in consequence movement of the joint is restricted, the toe is dragged on the

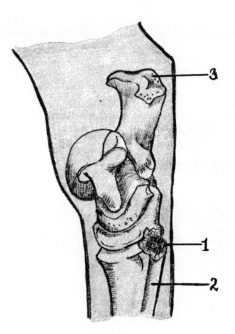

Fig. 25. Bones of Hock of
Horse, showing inside view
1. Spavin
2. Splint bone
3. Point of hock

ground, and the limb appears to swing outwards from the stifle.

A simple test consists of holding the limb up by the toe thereby forcibly flexing the joint. After about thirty seconds the toe is released and the animal trotted a few paces when lameness will be more evident if a spavin is present.

The term **Occult Spavin** applies to an inflammation of the same bones but only the articular surfaces are affected. Dragging of the toe in movement occurs but no external enlargement is found. There may be heat in the area and lameness does not diminish with exercise.

Treatment This is directed towards easing the pain through corrective shoeing and by promoting joint fusion, that is between the small bones of the hock and the head of the small splint bone. Rest is essential. Firing, either with point or line, preferably the former, will often hasten the process and result in partial or complete cure. A blister should follow firing and the animal be rested for at least a month.

Col. Codrington found that an iodine ointment, consisting of a 10 per cent iodine in a base of horse fat, applied daily, followed by the application of an infra-red lamp for ten to fifteen minutes, and continued for at least three weeks gave good results.

SPRAINS OF TENDONS AND LIGAMENTS

In view of the frequency with which strains of tendons and ligaments occur, especially in the race horse, and, to a lesser degree, the hunter, this subject is of considerable economic importance.

A tendon differs from a ligament both in texture and function, yet there are certain common factors which permit of their being grouped together.

Tendons The tendon is not an entity, but part of a muscle, the upper portion of which is flesh, known as the 'belly', and the lower portion strong fibrous strands, known as tendon.

The belly has much greater powers of contraction and expansion than the tendon and in consequence the former is less likely to strain than the latter.

The most common seat of sprained tendons is the flexors of the fore leg, running from the knee to the fetlock and foot, and in consequence these will now be dealt with in detail. In fact such injury is so frequent that loose terms, such as 'gone in front', 'broken down', 'developed a leg', etc., all refer to sprains of these tendons.

Cause The following are the main causes of strained tendons:
1. Fast work and fatigue when exhausted through unfitness;
2. Meeting a false or soft piece of ground when galloping;
3. Jumping dropped fences;
4. Slipping on treacherous ground;
5. Extravagant action of the excitable type;
6. Galloping too long on one track;
7. Long sloping pasterns;
8. Weakness of tendon fibres, due to heredity;
9. Conformation − (back at the knee).

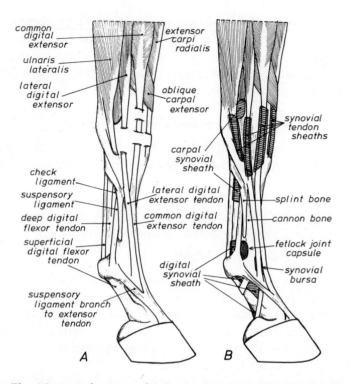

Fig. 26. Lateral aspect of right foreleg from the middle of the forearm down. A. Skin removed to show the muscle bellies above the knee joint and the relationships of their tendons extending down across the knee and fetlock joints towards the foot. B. The position of various synovial structures diagrammatically illustrated by cross-hatching. The synovial tendon sheaths facilitate the movement of tendons in the region of joints. Due to their subcutaneous position these synovial structures are liable to injury.

After considering the above causes it will be appreciated that the first six can be considered collectively as any influence which brings about a sudden and excessive stretching of a muscle before the upper resilient portion has had time to react, or is slow in doing so, due to fatigue. Normally, the upper fleshy portion acts as a buffer to the tendon and takes any shock, providing it is prepared and fit to receive that shock.

Excessively sloping pasterns and hereditary weakness of tendon fibres are both obvious causes.

Symptoms As symptoms will vary according to the extent of the injury and the tendons affected, a study of the sketch of these parts will help in identifying the different structures named in the following description.

Slight strain may affect the sheath and fibres of the superficial tendon only, resulting in heat and a small amount of swelling. There may be little or no lameness, but if the leg is picked up and slight pressure applied down this tendon with the finger and thumb, some pain will be evidenced. It must be remembered that slight pressure only must be applied, as a sound horse will flinch if the tendon is pinched hard.

A more severe strain with rupture of some of the fibres will cause a considerable amount of swelling along the whole length of the tendon. Lameness will be present and there will be acute pain on pressure with the fingers.

Rupture of any tendon in this area usually occurs about midway between knee and fetlock, resulting in an enlarged area, which can be felt easily when the leg is picked up and the tendon is relaxed. When standing at the side of a horse this enlargement may be seen, hence the term 'bowed tendon'.

Lastly, a complete breakdown occurs when the superficial and deep tendons are ruptured, with so much swelling that neither can be identified. There is acute lameness, the fetlock is dropped, and pain is evident from sweating and blowing.

Treatment There is considerable divergence of opinion as to the treatment of strained tendons. Col. Codrington suggested the application of hot poultices of antiphlogistine or kaolin immediately and firmly bandaged, this treatment being continued daily for at least a week to relieve pain and congestion. This stage is to be followed by cold water treatment, half an hours hosing two or three times a day to further reduce the inflammation and help in contracting the

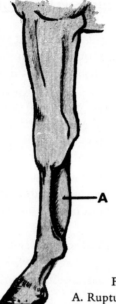
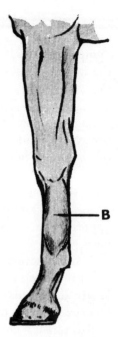

Fig. 27. Fore Legs
A. Ruptured Tendon
B. Sprained Suspensory Ligament

stretched tendon. Other authorities have recommended immediate bandaging, as tight as can be pulled, aiming at eliminating any possibility of tendon thickening or bowing. These authorities maintain that such features are enhanced should heat be applied without pressure.

Should bandaging be favoured this must be employed as soon as possible before any exudation has become solidified in the tissues. The bandaging must also be correctly applied with cotton wool or wadding arranged beneath the bandage to distribute pressure evenly. The bandage should be removed after 48 hours and the area massaged for some time. Hand-rubbing and massage are particularly useful in sprains to improve circulation in the part and prevent the formation of adhesions between parts by organization of exuded inflammatory fluid. The bandage should be replaced and massaging and rebandaging repeated every morning and evening for a week.

A further component of either treatment is that a wedge heel shoe may be used for the first ten to fourteen days to throw more weight on the toe and so relieve the tendon. However, prolonged treatment with wedges will induce the contraction of the tendons so that their replacement by tips in the later stages of recovery is indicated to encourage the tendons to remain less contracted.

Corticosteroid injections may also be administered by a veterinary surgeon, but cortisone may give rise to excessive fibrous tissue formation in and around tendons rendering subsequent adhesions and contractions more likely.

As soon as the heat and soreness have left the part gradual and gentle exercise may be commenced. Rest is generally essential in the early stages of some injuries but if prolonged for too long a period it allows the inflammatory exudate to stagnate. The tissue exudate during inflammation spreads into neighbouring tissues and if it is allowed to coagulate it may transform into granulation tissue and the surfaces in contact will adhere. If the granulation is undisturbed it will become organized and an adhesion will form which is impossible to separate. Because adhesions bind structures together and ultimately contract they do serious harm by limiting movement. Injuries to the superficial and deep flexor tendons must receive treatment which incorporates exercise. Initially, after the acute inflammatory stage has passed, this exercise can be produced passively by hand-rubbing and massage and also by electrotherapy, passing electric currents into the muscle tissues. Owing to the importance of muscular contraction and relaxation in promoting circulation and aiding removal of fluid exudate the stimulation of muscles presents a method of treatment not only for injured muscles and tendons but also for other tissues because muscular action improves the circulation through a wide area.

We can summarize by saying that a limited period of rest is essential following which slow walking work may be given. The former practice of giving six months to a year rest is not advisable as this long rest will allow the adhesions, which normally form in any inflammatory process, to become permanent.

Col. Codrington also recommended that at the end of a month a blister can be applied. One must not forget to apply a supporting bandage to the sound leg, seeing that it will be carrying most of the weight, especially in the early stages. Failure to do this may result in damage to the sound leg. The same thing applies in blistering, both legs being treated.

After blistering the patient can be turned out the following day and rested completely for six to eight weeks. But blistering and rest may well increase the possibilities of adhesion although the actual damaged tissue may benefit. The skin thickening produced by blistering may have a beneficial effect since it will act as a permanent bandage. However, it may constrict and so reduce the normal circulation that nutrition of the part is reduced.

Col. Codrington also recommended firing the horse in cases of appreciable breakdown after the leg has recovered from the first blister. As to the method used, it was Col. Codrington's opinion that line firing is much more efficient than point firing and the actual cautery is better than the use of strong acids.

Firing produces acute inflammation leading to loss of action. Owing to the pain and destruction of tissues by actual burns the horse rests the part as much as possible leading to congestion. It is difficult to see how this can have any appreciable beneficial effects on resolution of the strain. As a long-term method of treatment following the acute inflammatory stage, massage, bandaging, electrotherapy and short wave therapy are definitely preferable to blistering and firing.

Ligaments Although a ligament is made of hard fibres, like a tendon, it differs in that it has no upper resilient portion or belly and is much less elastic. Its main function is either to hold one or more bones together, or to act as a support to a joint.

The Suspensory Ligament This ligament is attached to the

the back of the cannon bone in a groove made by the latter and the two splint bones, and just above the sesamoid bones it splits into four strands. The two front strands wind round the fetlock joint and join the extensor tendon in front of the pastern, and the hind strands are attached to the sesamoid bones. Its function is to hold the fetlock joint in its suspended position, as its name implies. To a lesser extent it will act as a support to the tendons.

This ligament is not often subject to sudden strain, except when the tendons rupture, and in consequence damage to it is not usually a primary condition in the same sense as a sprained tendon. The usual cause is concussion from fast work on hard surfaces, or from general wear in the aged horse, and in consequence, it develops slowly.

Symptoms Should a sprain occur in conjunction with a rupture of the tendons, diagnosis may be difficult in the initial stages, owing to the great amount of swelling of the whole area. Any treatment of the injured tendons will also have some effect upon the suspensory ligament.

When the ligament is strained as a result of concussion or wear, inflammation and swelling may incorporate the tendons, but if the leg is examined carefully the outline of the latter can be felt, and in any case there will be no 'bow'.

Lameness is not present as such but the stride is shortened.

Treatment of the acute case associated with rupture of the tendons will be similar to that used for the latter.

Where the sprain is not associated with tendon troubles, fomentations of hot water, followed by kaolin poultices, may be used for the first week to reduce the initial inflammation. During this time the animal should be rested and all concentrated food withheld. The application of bandages is also a useful treatment either with the poultices or without. In mild cases once the inflammation has subsided a blister may be applied and the animal turned out for a month, preferably bandaged. After this the horse can commence steady work. Long rest, as in the case of sprained tendons, is quite unnecessary.

Finally, a word of warning regarding the possibility of swollen legs arising from causes other than from strain. Swelling of the fore legs may occur through infection from a wound caused by brushing or a punctured wound from a thorn, or even a pricked sole. Swelling occurs and the lesion may be mistaken for a sprained tendon. The main differences are:

Sprained Tendon	*Swelling from Infection*
1. Swelling affects the whole cannon.	Swelling is usually more on the inside or outside of the cannon, depending on the position of the wound.
2. Pain on pressure.	There may be no pain on pressure, but after pressing the imprint of one's finger remains.
3. Acute lameness.	Slight lameness.
4. Possible 'bow'.	No 'bow'.

The Check Ligament This ligament is a short structure starting at the back of the knee and extending half way down the cannon bone where it is joined to the deep flexor tendon. It acts as a support for the deep tendon.

This ligament may be strained when it is called upon to support extra weight through the muscular portion of the deep flexor being in a state of fatigue, or its failure to react to a sudden false step. Strain may occur without any of the other tendons being affected and is evidenced by a swelling on either side of the leg, extending from the back of the knee to the point where it joins the deep tendon.

Treatment Whether a primary condition or in conjunction with strain of other structures, rest is essential. If the sprain is slight a working blister may effect a cure, but if appreciable the tendons will be affected and the treatment will be common to both. A supporting bandage should be applied for two or three weeks and the horse confined to its stall for a month. In the acute stages corticosteroids may be injected to relieve the inflammation.

Curb A curb is the name given to a strain of the ligament which binds the bone forming the point of the hock to the top of the cannon bone. The swelling denoting curb can be seen when the hock is viewed from the side (see illustration).

If the head of the splint bone is unduly large an enlargement may be seen at the seat of the curb, but on examination this 'swelling' will be found to be hard and present on both limbs, whereas a curb is softer and usually occurs on one limb.

Sickle-shaped hocks are said to be most susceptible to strain of the curb ligament, but well-shaped hocks are not immune.

In the initial stages there may be lameness, but it is slight and of short duration.

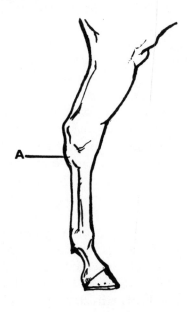

Fig. 28. A. Curb

Treatment Curb occurs most frequently in young horses and those that have not been doing well and are not fit. Most curbs resolve as the horse matures and no treatment is required.

Light firing and blistering will bring about a permanent cure and in fact most knowledgeable purchasers will not attach any importance to curby hocks, providing they have been fired.

In the case of a show horse firing is out of the question and a mild blister may be adequate. Should a trace of thickening be left, light rubbing with castor oil, followed by twenty to thirty 'strokes' over the part daily with a deer bone, will usually remove all traces after two to three weeks.

Stringhalt The term Stringhalt describes the action of the hind legs when a horse shows a sudden exaggerated flexion of the hock in one or both limbs, bringing them to the ground with a snap. It is seen when the animal moves from side to side in the stable, or when moved forwards from the standing position.

Very often stringhalt symptoms may be shown for a while and then be absent for a period. Later the jerky action and the snap of the foot may reappear and persist or be followed by another period of normal action.

Many theories have been put forward as to the cause of the condition, but they all lack positive proof. It is safe to say that the cause is of nervous origin. An operation can be performed which may alleviate and even abolish stringhalt, but as the effect on efficiency is not marked, surgical interference is not necessary in the great majority of cases.

Treatment No treatment is of much use but steps can be taken to alleviate the ill effects of excessive concussion since the foot is brought to the ground with some force. These measures will mainly be concerned with alterations to the shoes such as the addition of thick leather soles.

Where a hunter is badly affected his jumping capabilities do not appear to be impaired when 'going on' at a fence, but he is not keen on jumping from a standstill. One of the greatest of all 'chasers' was affected with very marked stringhalt.

Generally speaking, the condition is progesssive up to a point, after which it is stationary.

Some horses will only show the condition for the first few strides, or only occasionally when moved from side to side in the stable.

Shivering This is a disease arising from some abnormality or disfunction of the nervous system. The nerve supply to groups of muscles is interfered with and the muscles become unco-ordinated in action. It may be observed in any part of the body, but the back and hind limbs are the parts most frequently affected.

Nothing may be noticed when the animal is standing still, or in motion, but if asked to back or turn over quickly in the stable the tail may 'cock' and quiver, a hind limb may be snatched up and held in the air, and to avoid losing his balance, the horse will hop quickly on the other leg.

If asked to back, the horse will perhaps move its forelegs back a stride, but leave the hind legs in the same place. The back will be arched and only after difficulty, as though the animal is frightened to move the hind legs, will the latter be moved one stride in a snatchy manner.

As a rule, the condition is progressive and will eventually result in wasting of the muscles of the hind limbs.

Affected horses are loath to lie down, especially in the restricted area of a stall or box. Probably this is due to the instinctive fear that they will have difficulty in rising. To avoid this danger many horses have learnt to sit on the edge of the manger or on a strap or board placed across the end of their stall.

Synovial Enlargements When we mentioned joints in section one the synovial joint was introduced, being a joint enclosing a cavity into which a fluid (synovia) is secreted by a surrounding synovial membrane. As well as joints other structures are also possessed of a synovial secreting membrane to assist in the alleviation of compression and reduction of friction during movement, such structures as synovial bursae and synovial sheaths.

A **synovial bursa** is a sack, the inner walls of which are lined by a delicate membrane containing cells which secrete a fluid. When the sack is full the pressure of the fluid on these secreting cells stops further formation. Where a tendon, ligament or muscle passes over a bone, these sacks are interposed between the two structures as a buffer to avoid damage to either.

Through excessive pressure of the ligament, or tendon, the walls may become stretched, in which case a greater quantity of fluid will be required to fill the enlarged space and cause sufficient pressure on the secreting cells to stop or control production of the fluid. Inflammation and the subsequent

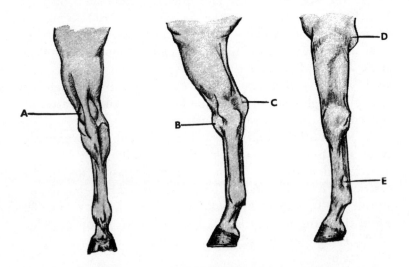

Fig. 29. Enlargements of synovial structures (bursae, sheaths and joint capsules).

A. Thoropin   C. Capped hock
B. Bog spavin   D. Capped elbow
                E. Wind gall

increase in fluid production may arise due to external violence such as falls.

Examples of these enlarged bursae may be seen at the point of the hock — **capped hock**, at the point of the elbow — **capped elbow**, and on either side of the withers — **lumpy withers** (if unattended to, leading to **fistulous withers**).

A **synovial sheath** is simply a bursa which is wrapped completely around a tendon so that the tendon slides up and down within this lubricated sheath. These tendon sheaths are found in the lower parts of the limbs where the long tendons of the muscles from the forearm and second thigh pass down across knee or hock and cannon and fetlock.

Examples of distended tendon sheaths may be seen where the deep flexor tendon passes over the back of the hock — **thoropin**, and at the back of the fetlock — **windgalls**.

Finally the **synovial joint capsules** themselves may be invaded by inflammatory germs or receive a violent blow and secrete excessive amounts of fluid into the joint causing visible swelling, as in **bog spavin**.

Treatment From the above description of the cause of these enlarged synovial structures, it is obvious that treatment should be directed towards exerting an artificial pressure on them, and thus restricting the amount of fluid formed, to allow the walls to contract.

In the case of wind galls constant pressure bandages may reduce them, but blistering is usually the most efficient. The latter acts by pressure from the thickened skin. However, it is probably best not to interfere with windgalls since they very seldom cause lameness and are a common occurence in old horses. Only if they become very large and interfere with joint action should they be treated.

Trusses designed to cause pressure on the enlarged synovial structures in cases of thoropin, bog spavin, and capped hocks, have been used, but as they must be taken off for exercise, the action is not constant and therefore unsatisfactory. Syphoning off the fluid with a hypodermic needle and injecting one of the Cortisone preparations into the bursa will reduce the swelling considerably, and in some cases the wall will contract back to normal. Should the swelling have existed for some time Cortisone treatment is not so satisfactory. All things considered it is probably best in the case of bog spavin or thoropin, provided that no lameness is present, to leave the swellings alone and not resort to any treatment which might well aggravate the condition.

Capped elbow is rather different in that the cause is usually due to pressure from the shoe when lying down. A bad or uneven floor is another cause. A sausage boot (named on account of its shape) strapped above the fetlock or around the pastern will prevent the foot from coming into contact with the elbow, and if applied when the enlargement is small, the swelling may subside. If, on the other hand, the skin has been broken and the bursa infected, surgical removal is necessary.

In the case of the poll, the bursa affected is the one interposed between the spine bone, just behind the ears, and the large ligament which comes from the withers and is attached to the top of the skull. The initial cause of the enlargement of the bursa is direct injury and frequently the skin is broken. Because serious complications may result, expert advice should be sought at once.

Pinches from the saddle on either side of the highest part of the withers may cause considerable trouble and incapacitate a horse for some time. As bruising occurs in these cases, a poultice, preferably of kaolin, should be applied for two to three days. The horse may be ridden after this, providing one can be certain that no further pressure will be applied. A thick numnah, with large holes cut over the seat of bruising, may be used to avoid further pressure. Rugs should also be cut away as they tend to slip backwards and exert considerable and constant pressure on this area. This pressure alone may be the cause of the initial damage and it will certainly aggravate an existing condition. Providing this is done no further treatment should be necessary.

Dropped Elbow This condition is caused by paralysis of the nerve controlling the muscles of the elbow. Such paralysis may occur as a result of over stretching the limb when falling or from the fracture of the first rib.

Treatment Little or no direct treatment is of any avail in view of the fact that the nerves affected, being in the 'arm pit' are inaccessible. Time is the main factor.

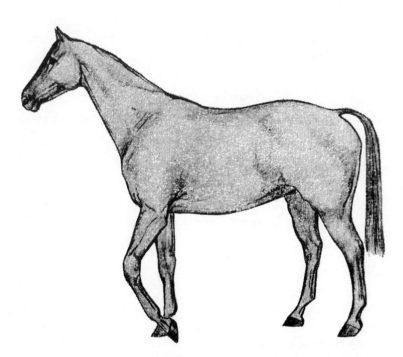

Fig. 30. Dropped Elbow or Radial Paralysis of the left forelimb showing the typical stance which is diagnostic of the condition: Elbow dropped lower than normal, knee and fetlock joints flexed, toe rested on the ground or in some cases the wall of the foot contacts the ground. The limb cannot be advanced and no weight is borne upon the leg the muscles becoming flaccid and soft.

Massage of the paralysed muscles for an hour or so at a time may be useful and electrical stimulation of the muscles to simulate normal muscle action can be tried. Light exercise is also useful but if no improvement occurs within six weeks destruction must be considered.

Should the callous formed as a result of fracture of the first rib incorporate or cause considerable pressure on the nerve the chances of recovery are slight. On the other hand should the nerve be stretched only recovery may occur in a few weeks.

If the limb is placed in the normal position and the patient can stand on it this is an indication that there is a reasonable chance of recovery.

FAULTY ACTION

Horses, who in their paces hit a fore or hind limb with the hoof or shoe of the opposite foot, are said to brush. The point of contact varies and a terminology has been devised to describe and identify the site and type of injury.

Speedy Cutting The point of contact is just underneath the knee. It occurs in horses with very high action, such as hackneys.

Brushing The injury is inflicted round about the bulb of the fetlock or the top of the foot.

These conditions are almost always found in young animals shod for the first time, old and weak horses that are overworked, at the beginning of the training season when the horse is out of condition, or at the end of a long hard ride when the horse is tired out. Very occasionally it is the result of faulty shoeing and also in a fit horse it occurs usually in the narrow-chested animal, with, or without, turned out toes.

In the case of a horse with straight action, the movement of the legs from the fetlock down describe parallel lines, but where the toes are turned out, the feet describe converging lines in action Thus, when the toe is brought forward, it hits the opposite fetlock.

As suggested by the reasons for brushing occurring given above, treatment is normally straightforward. Unfit horses should be given lighter work until fit; horses that are tired should be driven slowly, etc. If these measures fail efforts at prevention must be directed towards straightening the action and this can be achieved by shoeing. The outside branch of the shoe should be one-eighth of an inch thicker than the inner, and the toe clip a half inch inwards from the central position.

In most cases brushing will be cured after three to four shoeings.

Dishing This term applies to an animal whose lower fore limb is thrown outwards in movement and is more often seen in common bred horses. Horses with such action are liable to be unsafe in deep going.

This action can be partially and in some cases completely rectified by shoeing with a thick-toed shoe, so as to increase the weight at that point.

Loss of Fore-Leg Action Loss of action in front can be caused by incorrect shoeing, such as dumping the toe, failure to open the heels, resulting in a contracted hoof, and lack of frog pressure. It may be occasioned by injury or disease in the interior of the foot. Circulatory failure, such as congestion, is a frequent cause. 'Pottery action' is a common term used to describe these cases, in which the stride is shortened.

It is seen in cases of Navicular disease and Pedal Ostitis, where the cause is a chronic congestion of the feet, and may result from fast work on hard roads.

Forging This is the term used when the hind foot hits the fore foot. The toe of the hind shoe hits the inner edge of the fore shoe.

It occurs most often in heavy horses when they are shod with extravagant 'champhered' show shoes. It is not observed so often in the lighter horses. It may be caused by weakness in the young horse and may disappear as the animal gains strength and muscular control.

To prevent forging the hind shoe should be set back a little under the toe and the inner edge of the fore shoe should be concaved.

Fractures In spite of the risks that horses are subjected to, either in the field of racing or hunting, fractures of bones are not common. Bones are constructed to carry normal weight, stress and strains, but a false step, whereby the whole weight of the body is thrown on a portion of the bone, may be the cause of a fracture.

A good example of this can be quoted. A horse was driven at a small fence with a ditch on the take-off side. The horse refused, was held at the fence, and eventually sprawled across it. The result was a fracture of both sesamoid bones, due to over extension of the fetlock joint.

Symptoms Usually fractures are suspected when the onset of lameness is sudden and pain so acute that no weight can be placed on the affected limb. When a long bone, such as the cannon or radius in the fore limb, and the cannon, or tibia in the hind, is fractured, diagnosis is comparatively simple, owing to the distortion of the limb. Even slight manipulation of the limb will cause acute pain, and possible a diagnostic grating, caused by the friction of the fractured ends on each other, can be felt and sometimes heard.

When a shorter bone is fractured, such as that of the pastern, there may be little distortion of the limb, but pain will be acute and slight manipulation of the limb from the foot will cause considerable distress.

When sudden acute lameness occurs, with or without distortion of the limb, coupled with general disturbance, such as blowing and sweating, it is wise to suspect a fracture and seek professional advice and aid immediately.

If the diagnosis is in doubt, an X-ray will be of great value.

Treatment It has been held against the Veterinary Profession that no attempt is made to treat fractures, but the people who make such a complaint do not appreciate the reason for the apparent inaction.

When a long bone, such as the cannon or tibia, is fractured transversely, unless the limb can be completely immobilised, there is little hope of a satisfactory fusion. It is almost impossible to provide rigid immobilisation in a large animal. On the other hand, if the fracture is longitudinal without any misplacement of the parts, complete resolution may be possible. It must be remembered that when a bone is fractured new bone is laid down at the site of injury. Should the new repair bone tissue affect a joint or interfere with movement of a ligament or tendon, complete recovery is impossible.

Should the patient be a mare or stallion and be required for breeding, some degree of ambulatory disfunction or lameness is of little account.

Fractures in horse bones repair just as readily as do the bones of any other animal, including man. Horses that work or race have to be sound in action, otherwise the owners and riders or drivers stand in peril of prosecution for cruelty. A horse which has some ambulatory disability cannot be used. Because of the almost insuperable difficulty in providing for complete immobilisation, perfect functional results cannot be guaranteed and, for economic reasons, the owners prefer to cut their losses and destroy. The sort of repair which is considered good, yet leaves a man a cripple, would be of no value in a horse.

The author has known of fractures of the pelvis, the small bone behind the knee, cannon bone and pastern recovering and the animal winning races afterwards, but in each case there was no misplacement of the fractured pieces and the resultant callous did not interfere with the movement of any joint.

When estimating the possibility of recovery from fractures, the Veterinary Surgeon will base his prognosis on many factors.

CHAPTER TEN

Digestive Disorders

Teeth For correct functioning of the digestive system the food must be suitably prepared in the mouth. Any irregularity of the teeth may interfere with efficient mastication, the main reason being as follows: because the upper jaw is wider than the lower, and the movement is from side to side, the inner edges of the teeth of the lower jaw and the outer edges of the upper jaw are not worn and remain as sharp points. These needle-like portions may lacerate the inner cheek or tongue during movement, thus causing incomplete mastication and consequent malnutrition. Symptoms of these sharp edges existing are:

Quidding-partly chewed hay will drop out of the mouth in balls.

The head is often held on one side when chewing and the movement of the jaws is cautious and restricted. Laceration of the tongue or cheek may be seen and the sharp edges can be felt.

These edges can be removed with a tooth rasp. To facilitate the use of the rasp and to avoid the tongue being damaged, the latter should be drawn out of the mouth on the opposite side and held lightly. Excessive rasping is the common error in this operation. As the needle edges only need removing, a few up and down movements of the rasp will usually suffice.

If the cheeks or tongue have been injured, the use of the rasp may cause increased soreness and in consequence it is advisable to prescribe a diet of sloppy food for a few days after the operation.

From injury, such as a kick, a molar may be broken. In such a case food will pass through the gap and collect between the cheek and teeth and may be seen from the outside as a bulge. This collected food will soon ferment and cause a strong foetid breath. Beyond removing the food once or twice a day nothing further can be done.

Lampas This term is applied to a condition in which the palate of the upper jaw, immediately behind the incisor teeth, becomes swollen. It is often seen about the time when the permanent teeth are erupting through the gums at 2½, 3½ and 4½ years.

Quite erroneously the condition has been considered to be a primary lesion, but in actual fact it is a symptom of indigestion, dietetic errors or the general falling off in condition which naturally occurs when teeth are being cut. If it appears in an older animal it may be a symptom of a more general systemic disease or malnutrition.

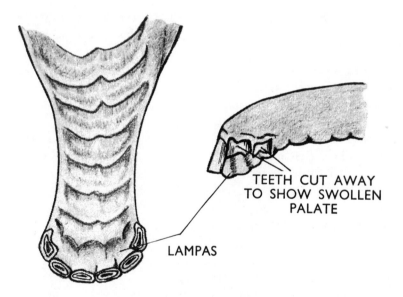

Fig. 31. Lampas
left　Upper jaw showing palate and inflamed area known as lampas
right　Upper jaw showing inflamed area of palate known as lampas
　　　　protruding below the level of tooth

Treatment In the old days, because the palate was swollen and protruded below the teeth, it was thought that pain from the friction of food on it caused lack of appetite. Actually, the lack of appetite is due to a deranged digestion and in consequence, treatment should be directed towards improving the general condition of the animal. If this is achieved the swelling will subside automatically. A useful corrective powder is as follows: Epsom Salts 8 oz.; Glucose 4 oz.; Bicarbonate of soda 2 oz.; Nitrate of Potash ½ oz. One tablespoonful to be given night and morning on dry food or in the drinking water for seven to ten days.

Choking This is a blockage of the tube down which food passes from the mouth to the stomach. The cause may be an apple, potato, or large piece of root, or a mass of dry food bolted by a tired but greedy feeder.

The symptoms are salivation, frequent attempts at swallowing, causing a gurgling sound, and at intervals the head is drawn in to the chest, the muscles of the neck are tensed and then the head is stretched out again. If one stands on the near side and observes the neck along the jugular groove, as the animal attempts to swallow a wave of movement can be seen ending in a gurgle, when the animal salivates and champs its jaws.

Treatment *At no time should any drench be given,* as it will most likely pass into the lungs with serious consequences. A lump of lard or butter should be smeared on the tongue and teeth. A little of either will pass into the food tube and so will assist the passage of the mass. Light massage down the jugular groove on the near side may assist.

If the condition is not relieved within half an hour expert advice must be sought.

Two notes of warning re this are:

a. Do not give a greedy feeder a dry feed when coming in from a long day for at least an hour — give a small drink and a little hay.

b. Do not offer water to a choking horse if you know the

obstruction is dry food, as it may well swell the mass and so aggravate the obstruction.

Diarrhoea There is little need to explain this condition, but the causes may be divided into Benign and Malignant Diarrhoea.

Benign cases may be due to:

a. Nervous reaction in an excitable animal;
b. Sudden surfeit of green fodder;
c. An overdose of a purgative;
d. An excess of fatty food, such as barley or clover hay;
e. Faulty teeth.

In every case the treatment is obvious.

Malignant Diarrhoea may be due to:

a. Without a temperature — slight inflammation of the bowel from irritant food, such as heated oats; and heavy worm infestation.
b. With temperature — enteritis due to infection.

If the cause is obvious the appropriate treatment, together with a diet of hay and bran for a few days, should effect a cure, but if the diarrhoea persists, advice should be taken as purging may be serious due to the withdrawal of large amounts of fluid from the body.

Constipation in a horse, coupled with loss of condition, is generally due to lack of tone of the bowel, due to a poor diet. It may also occur following a strong purgative, especially if the latter is not followed up with bran mashes for a few days after dosing.

In either case *the condition should be relieved with a laxative diet — grass and bran mashes, rather than resort to purgatives.*

Worms There are four main groups of worms infesting the equine as follows:

1. *Oxyuris* or Seat Worm.
2. *Ascaris* or Round White Worm.

3. *Dictyocaulus* or Lung Worm.
4. *Strongyle* or Red Worm.

Seat Worm This group rarely gives rise to any general symptoms except rubbing of the tail. Their presence is manifested by a yellowish white deposit around the anus and perineum.

Treatment A solution of 2 tablespoons epsom salts dissolved in 1 pint warm water and given as an enema, and repeated at intervals of a week for 3 doses will remove the egg laying females which collect in the rectum. The dock sponge should be disinfected frequently to prevent reinfection.

Round White Worm or *Ascaris* are the most common types found in the horse and donkey. They are 6 to 12 inches long, yellowish white, the thickness of a pocket diary pencil, and pointed at one end. Their presence in the adult has little general effect, but can cause considerable general disturbance in the young animal up to 3 years old.

Life Cycle The female lays eggs in the gut which are passed out in the droppings. Once on the pasture the eggs develop into an immature worm called a larva but these infective forms remain inside the protective egg shell until they are eaten by an animal. Once in the gut the eggs hatch and the larvae penetrate the intestinal wall and migrate throughout the internal organs to the lungs. They are then coughed up and swallowed finally returning to the gut where they develop into adult worms.

If present in large numbers they have been known to cause a blockage or even rupture of the gut and death in the young.

Symptoms Unless these worms are present in large numbers there is little general disturbance, a diagnosis being made only when they are seen in the droppings. There may be loss of condition in the young, staring coat and irregular bowel action, with the passage of a small quantity of fluid following a motion.

Treatment Aloes in a tasteless form given on a mash was

quite an effective treatment but it required several days of preparation with sloppy mashes to ensure a quick passage of the drug through the bowel. Aloes is, however, a powerful purgative and if used without due care or suitable preparation may well be dangerous owing to its violent and painful purging action on the bowel. In fact it is best not to use aloes when there is inflammation in the gut or when the horse is in a debilitated condition. Both of these situations may pertain in *Ascaris* infestation. Aloes has in fact been superseded by Piperazine Adipate which is more efficient, requires less preparation of the animal and is not associated with undue purging. As with Red Worm infestation periodic dosing to cope with the larvae which are constantly returning to the bowel is necessary. For control of pasture contamination see under Red Worms.

Dictyocaulus or Lung Worm The increase in popularity of the donkey and the blame attached to it for the spread of infestation to the horse, make it necessary to deal with this group of worms separately. They are round worms as are Oxyuris, Ascaris and Strongyle ·but with an important difference in their life cycle.

Life Cycle *a.* The adult male and female live in the bronchioles or breathing tubes of the lung. Eggs are laid in the mucous normally formed in these tubes and are coughed up into the throat. Some are expelled into the air and presumably perish but the majority are swallowed and eventually excreted by the gut. *b.* Within an hour or two of being excreted the eggs hatch into the first stage larva or immature worm. After 48 hours another moult occurs to a second stage larva, which in a minimum time of 6 to 7 days is considered to be 'infective' or 'ripe'. In other words larvae picked up before the second stage are ineffective. *c.* Once the ripe larvae have been swallowed they migrate through the tissues to the lung where, after certain changes, they become adults and commence another cycle.

The ripening of the larvae on pastures will be slowed down

considerably by very hot dry weather or extreme cold, but will be rejuvenated by warm humid climate. Frost does not kill the larvae. The time lapse from larvae to adult worm is normally about 6 weeks.

Tolerance to infestation appears to be far greater in the donkey than the horse, the result being that coughing is far less pronounced, and may even be absent, hence the mistaken idea that the donkey infests the horse.

Susceptibility Present evidence points to the hunter, pony and donkey being more susceptible than the thoroughbred, but this may prove to be due to fitness enabling an animal to overcome infestation either in the gut or during migration to the lung. This is on a par with practical evidence that Red Worm infestation is definitely adversely affected in development in fit, well fed animals.

Diagnosis The presence of a dry cough is by no means indicative of infestation with lung worms, but laboratory examination of faeces can reveal the larvae which will be an important fact in making a differential diagnosis. Expert opinion must be sought to establish whether other causes such as, *a.* A focus of infection left from infection with the influenza virus. *b.* An allergy to bedding or hay. *c.* Emphysema from poorly ventilated stables, or over stretching of the lungs from excessive exertion, are the contributory causes. However, if microscopic examination of faeces reveals the presence of egg laying females they must be eliminated.

Treatment Actual. Several drugs are effective against round worms generally but there is no specific remedy to compare with the vaccine so successfully used in cattle.

'Franocide' (diethylcarbamazine citrate) administered in the drinking water has claimed some success, but half an ounce of turpentine in half a pint of linseed oil given by stomach tube about twice weekly has also given good results. Treatment also consists of good nursing and nourishing foods.

Prevention. As land can only become infected from an animal, all imports of either horses or donkeys to an existing group of animals that are free, or on to 'clean' land, should be isolated until a laboratory examination of faeces reveals the presence or absence of larvae, and in the event of the former, appropriate treatment has been administered.

Only because the donkey can be infested without showing any cough is it so important to have any import tested before allowing it to run with other equines.

Finally, low lying wet pastures should be avoided where possible in late summer and autumn.

Red Worms The red worm, or stongyle, is the one that warrants the most attention, as it can be the cause of serious general disturbance and a heavy infestation in the young animal may cause death.

There are two main types of Red Worm or Strongyle,
a. The Large Strongyle about one inch long;
b. The Small Strongyle about one-quarter to two-thirds of an inch.

The life cycle of both is as follows:

The adult male and female worms live in the intestines, the female laying eggs which are passed out with the droppings. On the pasture or on wet bedding a young worm, called a larva, develops within the egg. Under ideal climatic conditions, moisture and warmth, the larva escapes from the egg and is capable of infecting a horse/pony. It creeps up the moist herbage and is eaten by the animal. Once having gained access to the intestines the larvae of the large strongyle penetrate the gut wall and migrate throughout the internal organs and blood vessels before returning to the intestines to develop into adult worms.

The larvae of the small strongyles develop in the gut wall and eventually return to the intestines to mature.

The adult large strongyles and some of the small species attach themselves to the gut wall and suck blood whilst the others live on the digested food in the gut.

Symptoms The first symptoms are a general loss of condition, anaemia, distended stomach and staring coat. The actions of the bowel are irregular, with a tendency to diarrhoea, and there is usually a strong sour smell, especially noticed where the animal is housed. If the droppings are examined carefully, especially after the week-end mash, the actual worms may be seen.

Microscopic examination of the fresh droppings for the presence of eggs may give some indication of the extent of infestation. This test is not too reliable, as the egg count may vary and is not always proportionate to the degree of infection.

The irregular action and the rancid smell of the droppings is due to irritation and may be inflammation of the bowel, caused by the worms actually embedding themselves in the bowel wall and interfering with the normal physiological function. The worms may be so numerous that on post mortem examination, if the bowel is held up to the light, it gives the appearance of having been fired at with a shot gun.

A more serious and usually fatal sequel occurs when the worm works its way from the bowel into one of the main arteries supplying the gut. It becomes embedded in the wall of the artery and the tissue reaction, which includes swelling, may close up the artery, thereby cutting off the blood supply to the bowel. If the occlusion be complete the immediate result is an acute colic and death. As a rule such acute disasters are seen in young animals.

The effects of red worm infestation vary according to the age and diet of an animal. Whatever medicaments are used, microscopic examination of the droppings will reveal the presence of eggs, even after severe dosing. In other words, the red worm can be considered as a permanent parasite in the bowel of a horse and treatment will reduce the count, but not eradicate the worm completely. This fact is of some importance in considering the theory that the extent of the infestation and the damage caused depends on the general health of the host. An animal's body can develop some degree of resistance to these parasites.

Should digestive disturbance occur due to poor pastures,

insufficient diet for the young growing animal, or excessive exposure in bad weather, the physiological function of the bowel is upset and the intestinal contents tend to an acid reaction, forming an ideal medium for the propagation of the worm.

A simple test to illustrate this last point is the addition of an alkali, to counteract the acidity, in the form of 2-3 tablespoons of bicarbonate of soda in a mash. The following day a large number of adult worms will be seen in the droppings.

Treatment Since the introduction of a drug called Thiabendazole, marketed under the name Equizole, the eradication of adult worms in the gut is much more efficient. Previous treatment with Phenothiazine or Oil of Chenopodium was reasonably efficient but they both had the disadvantage of causing toxic side effects on the animal, in some cases. Strongyles can build up a resistance to the continued use of phenothiazine or even thiabendazole, this can be overcome by using piperazine with either of them.

There are two methods of dosing with Thiabendazole:
a. Small daily doses or a larger weekly dose is given in the feed. This method reduced the rate of egg laying by the female, and those eggs that are laid are not fertile, thus pasture contamination is reduced. The great disadvantage of this system is that the adult worms are not eliminated and in consequence, a low count of eggs revealed in microscopic examination of faeces gives no indication of the number of adult worms causing damage to the gut.
b. A full dose given every six weeks will remove the adult worms in the gut.

One must realise that whatever drug is used only the adult worms in the gut will be eradicated, hence the necessity of periodic dosing to cope with the migrating larvae which are constantly returning to the gut to mature.

Finally, other than measures to control worm infestation in the animal, certain action is necessary to minimise re-infestation from contaminated pastures. During the summer droppings should be picked up daily seeing that the larvae will hatch from the egg and migrate on to the grass in twenty-four hours, whereas twice weekly in the winter is adequate. In the case of animals that are stabled the practice of heaping up the bedding under the manger should be avoided, as the larvae can creep up the damp straw and gain access to the manger and food.

Although rotation of pastures is a sound husbandry measure it is of doubtful use in worm control since a substantial decrease in the number of larvae takes a longer period of time than that for which a pasture could be rested practicably.

Harrowing is of doubtful value in that, although strong sun may kill some of the eggs and larvae, nevertheless it increases the area of pasture contaminated by them.

Colic means abdominal pain. The term is used by horsemen to describe pain arising in the stomach, or intestines, of a horse. The horse is more susceptible to abdominal pain than most animals for the following general reasons:

a. The lining membrane of a horse's bowel is particularly sensitive.

b. The stomach is comparatively small, so that, in the event of gorging, food will pass on into the bowel before it has been adequately treated by the digestive juices.

The exciting causes of colic can be classified as follows:

1. Incomplete mastication of food, due to faulty teeth, or bolting the food.
2. Irregularity in times of feeding and too long intervals between meals.
3. Poor quality foods — heated oats, old, or musty hay, or in the case of a greedy feeder, bedding straw.
4. Accidental access to wheat or barley.
5. Sudden change of food, e.g. from soft meadow to hard seed hay.
6. Excessive quantity of cold water when hot.

7. Overwork leading to ravenous feeding when tired.

8. Too little exercise coupled with full working feeds.

There are several different types of colic, but as their differentiation requires considerable diagnostic skill and experience, the various types can be dealt with collectively.

The signs and symptoms at the outset are very similar.

Symptoms The usual initial symptoms of colic, in order of appearance, are:

a. General uneasiness;

b. Looking back at the sides and kicking at the abdomen;

c. Pawing the ground with either fore leg;

d. Getting up and down;

e. When down, lying out fully stretched and groaning;

f. Attempts to pass water;

g. Passing small quantities of droppings;

h. On putting one's ear to the flank, little, or no movement of the bowel is heard;

i. Absence of any rise in temperature.

Providing that the symptoms do not become more violent and no complications arise, such a case generally responds to simple treatment. The rate of the pulse and the colour of the eye membranes help one to assess if the colic be serious or not. If the pulse rate does not exceed 45-50 and the eye membranes are not deeper in colour than a pale salmon pink, there is no cause for undue alarm.

Treatment *Expert assistance should be obtained whenever an attack persists for more than three hours.* In simpler cases treatment is directed towards relieving pain and lubricating the intestinal tract. Food should be withheld until any evidence of pain is no longer present. A slight attack of colic, whether due to excessive flatulence, or irritant material in the gut, will respond to a mild purgative, to which has been added a stimulant. The following, given as a drench, is quite effective: Kaolin emulsion 1 pint; Water ½ pint; Sal Volatile 2 tablespoons.

If possible, enemata of warm soapy water should be given

in large amounts, but large quantities of fluid should not be given by stomach tube.

While discussing the treatment of a mild colic, Col. Codrington gave a warning regarding the indiscriminate use of the so called 'Brown Drink' or other proprietary colic drinks. Usually the active principle in such a drink is chlorodyne or some opium compound, which 'deadens' pain by reducing the sensitivity of the nerves.

When dealing with the nervous system it was explained that all movement of voluntary and involuntary muscle was controlled by the nerve impulses, and as treatment of an uncomplicated colic should be directed towards promoting the action of the bowel and the removal of offending irritant material in the gut, any drug, such as chlorodyne, which slows down the nerve impulses and so reduces the activity of the bowel, is contra-indicated.

After drenching, straw should be laid across the back and a jute rug put on inside out, to avoid the blanket lining getting wet from sweat. Pain usually occurs in waves and when acute the animal can be walked slowly to avoid it throwing itself about, but rested when the pain subsides.

Should the purgative *cum* stimulant drench have no effect within an hour, *a Veterinary Surgeon should be called without delay*. Should one not be available at once a repeat of the first drench may be given, as it will not aggravate or hinder subsequent treatment by an expert.

Because there appears to be some confusion regarding the condition known as 'twisted gut', a word or two will not be amiss here.

Normally the gut is suspended from the back along its entire length by a thin membrane called the mesentery. This mesentery is fan shaped and the gut lies in coils. Should a portion of this mesentery be torn away from the gut there is nothing to prevent the free portion revolving on itself, and in fact, this is what happens. Circulation is disturbed and there may be acute and serious pain. A twist of the gut means death to the patient.

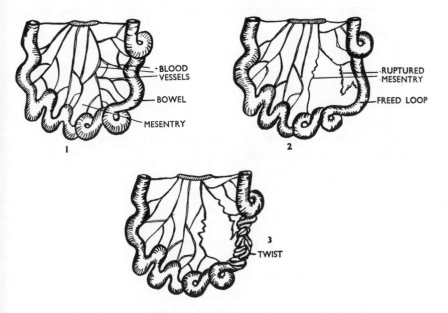

Fig. 32. Twisted Gut: sequence of events resulting in twist
1. Normal portion of gut suspended in abdomen by mesentery
2. Portion of mesentery ruptured leaving loop of bowel free to revolve on itself
3. Freed loop twisted

There are many theories regarding the cause of a twist, viz:

a. A horse may slip and if a portion of the bowel is heavily loaded with food, the mesentery may rupture from the sudden movement.
b. Violent purgatives causing excessive bowel movement against an impacted mass of food.
c. The horse throwing himself to the ground in the intitial violent stage of colic.

Rolling during an attack of colic is not mentioned as a cause of twist. Most experienced Veterinary Surgeons do not subscribe to this view. In the past this idea had much support and an animal was walked about, sometimes for hours, to avoid rolling. An occasional short walk may be beneficial to assist in the general movement of the gut and prevent the horse from throwing himself about, but constant exercise will exhaust the horse and his powers of recovery will be weakened.

Symptoms In the initial stages a 'Twisted Gut' is not easy to diagnose, but typical symptoms appear eventually, as follows:

a. The pulse becomes more rapid and is very thready.

b. Profuse patchy sweating occurs.

c. The animal becomes violent.

d. The eye membranes are very deep red.

e. The temperature rises up to 104° or 105°.

f. Constant movement of the bowel may be heard.

g. Breathing is greatly accelerated.

h. On examination per rectum, the anus will be found to be very tight and the bowel tightly contracted.

Treatment There is no treatment and the animal should be destroyed directly a definite diagnosis has been made.

On post mortem examination the twist may be found to be so tightly coiled that it is impossible to undo it.

Occasionally one is met on arrival at a case of colic with the words 'I think it's her water', and I would like to explain the reason for this once popular opinion.

The horse's bowel is very sensitive and the offending cause of the colic may result in excessive irritation of the nerve endings and the gut may go into a spasm. As the muscles of the bladder are supplied by the same group of nerves as the bowel, the muscle of the neck of the bladder is affected similarly, preventing the passing of water. Once the spasm has been relieved, the muscle controlling the neck of the bladder will be one of the first to relax and allow water to be passed. Thus, because the passing of water heralded a relief of symptoms, one can understand why a temporary failure to pass water freely was considered to be the actual cause of colic.

CHAPTER ELEVEN

Respiratory Diseases

NOSE, THROAT AND LUNG INFECTIONS

The horse is particularly susceptible to nose, throat and lung infections. Lack of fresh air and sudden change in temperature play an important contributory part in causing coughs, colds, pneumonia and emphysema. Evidence supporting this contention can be seen in those parts of the world where horses are kept in badly ventilated stables, for the incidence of emphysema is very high.

Horses that are brought in from grass and placed in badly ventilated stables frequently develop coughs and colds.

Always remember that if warmth is required it is best to rely on clothing, but leave windows and the top door open.

COUGHS

Coughing is a symptom of irritation in the membrane lining the larynx or the upper part of the windpipe and is the cardinal symptom in all inflammatory conditions of the throat. However, it may result from any of the following:
1. A direct irritation to an inflamed throat from infection or injury;
2. Irritation of lung, or its covering membrane, the pleura, from infection;
3. Irritation of the breathing tubes of the lung from worm infestation;
4. Reflex irritation of the throat from stomach disorder.

A comparative table is perhaps the best method for quick reference as to differentiation.

On analysis of this table it will be seen that a stomach cough differs from throat infections mainly in that there are no swollen glands, temperature, or nasal discharge, and a lung

	Cough due to inflamed throat from infection	*Cough due to lung or pleura irritation from infection*	*Reflex stomach irritation*
Cause	Sea journey. Hot, badly ventilated stable from grass.	Chill from exposure.	Bad fodder, or too quick change from grass to dry feed.
Symptoms			
Noise	Soft, fluid, short.	Longer, soft and painful.	Short, hollow and hard.
Nasal Discharge ..	Clear to slightly opaque.	Thick white.	Nil.
Temperature ..	Perhaps 1° rise.	3°–4° or more rise.	Normal.
Breathing Rate.. ..	Normal.	Increased.	Normal.
Noises heard when applying ear to ribs	Nil.	Wheezing sounds.	Nil.
Throat glands	Swollen.	May be slightly swollen.	Normal.

condition is evidenced mainly by rise in temperature and quickened breathing.

Treatment In the case of a simple cough, with little rise in temperature, but slight swelling of the glands behind the lower jaw and underneath it, ensure plenty of fresh air, a laxative diet and a paste or electuary containing Potassium Chlorate to allay the irritation. Gentle exercise in hand is helpful.

A paste containing glycerine and M & B powder may be used and the head steamed with Friar's Balsam.

Where a cough is accompanied by several degrees rise in temperature and quickened breathing, pneumonia is most likely the cause. Rugs, bandages, and hood should be applied and Veterinary attention sought at once, as timely treatment with antibiotics will often bring about a rapid cure.

Stomach Cough This is often a harsh dry cough, which occurs at exercise or in the stable. Because it is due usually to digestion, all concentrated foods should be withheld and hay, cut grass, mashes, and a corrective medicine given for a week. The following will be found useful: Epsom Salts ½ lb.; Bicarbonate of Soda 2 oz.; Potassium Nitrate ½ oz. One tablespoon of mixture in food or drinking water morning and night.

Equine Influenza For many years a highly infectious condition occurs annually, commencing about March and continuing throughout the summer, the main symptom being a cough. This condition was loosely referred to as Epidemic Cough, but is now known as Equine Influenza. It is caused by a virus, and spreads via the atmosphere, as well as contact. Except for a distressing cough, loss of appetite, depression, and a slight clear nasal discharge, there is often little else to be noted. The active infection runs its course in seven to ten days, but the cough persists for weeks especially when the animal is worked. Occasionally a case runs a high temperature together with a yellow tinge to the gums, inner surface of the lips, and the membranes on the inside of the eyelids. This symptom may be due to the fact that infection is centred in the liver and/or gall bladder. None of the known antibiotics appears to have any beneficial effect, except possibly terramycin, but there is a preventive vaccine, which gives some degree of immunity lasting for about a year. The first injection should be given to foals of about three months and the second three months later. A single 'booster' dose is then administered to yearlings and then annual injections for the active life of the horse.

Influenza-like symptoms can also be produced by viruses outside the influenza group, e.g. rhinopneumonitis. Obviously the influenza vaccine will afford no protection against these infections.

In all cases concentrated foods should be discontinued, except possible 1 or 2 lb. boiled barley in a mash, for the first seven to ten days, after which a period at grass where possible.

Lung Worm Infestation Infestation of the lungs in equines by a type of round worm known as Dictyocaulus or Lung Worm frequently causes coughs in horses and to a lesser degree in donkeys. This subject has been dealt with under the heading 'Worms' in the chapter on digestive disorders.

Sinus Infection The skull contains several air spaces known as sinuses. There are three in number and each connects with the other. One is connected with the nose. Infection of either or all these cavities may follow injury to the bones forming them. In the case of one sinus the bony sockets of two of the molar teeth protrude into the cavity. Should injury or infection of these teeth occur their sockets may become involved which in turn may result in an infection of the sinus.
Symptoms The main symptom is a nasal discharge, greyish in colour evident in one nostril only. If the bone is diseased the discharge may be tinged with blood. The glands of the head are not swollen and there is no noise heard in breathing as is evident in nose and throat infections. If the condition has

existed for some time the bone or bones of the face forming the cavity may be distorted.

Treatment Drainage is essential and this can be effected by opening the cavity at its lowest extremity. This operation is not always successful, especially if the bone is diseased.

Emphysema A horse suffering from this condition is commonly known as 'Broken Winded'. Occasionally the term is applied rather loosely to any unsoundness of a horse's wind.

To understand the condition properly one should consider first the action of breathing.

The diaphragm is drawn back, thus creating a partial vacuum in the chest, the lungs expand and fill with air. The lungs, which contain much elastic tissue, then contract and together with the forward pushing movement of the diaphragm, the air is expelled.

If the lungs become over distended, some of the elastic tissue may be damaged, so that they lose their contracting powers and do not collapse completely. Damage to the elastic tissue involves the breaking down of some of the walls of the air cells. These air cells are lined by the membrane through which the oxygen in the air comes into contact with the blood. Damage to the walls of the cells means that the area provided for this interchange is much reduced and to compensate, the breathing rate has to be increased. It is also laboured because of the loss of elastic recoil. Overstrain, when unfit, such as excessive galloping, causing the lungs to expand suddenly to allow of a greater intake of oxygen, will cause this. Broken wind also often follows pneumonia or some bronchitic condition, and it has been suggested that lung worm infestation may cause it.

With a view to forcing the residual air out of the damaged lungs, the stomach muscles are brought into play, thus producing a double respiratory movement on expiration. When the abdominal muscles contract forcibly, they force the bowels forward against the diaphragm, which further reduces the size of the lung cavity.

Symptoms At the end of expiration, a line, which varies according to the degree of broken wind, can be seen on the abdomen, stretching from the level of the stifle forward. This is caused by the tightening of the muscles which contract the bowel cavity. It may not be very obvious until the animal is exerted, but a typical short hollow cough may precede this symptom. The cough may occur at any time at work or at rest, and often it is accompanied by the passing of wind.

As time goes on the cough becomes more persistent and the double expiration is quite obvious in the stomach muscles at the flank, breathing is laboured, and a wheezing sound will be heard, like that observed in an asthmatical man.

The cause of the cough may be temporary air hunger, or it may be due to spasm of the muscle tissue in the damaged lung. Some think that it may be due to some nerve disfunction.

Treatment Once the condition is well established, there is little one can do to effect a cure. A considerable amount of relief can be effected by reducing hay to a minimum, or replacing by oat straw, feeding more concentrates, and avoiding fast work.

The feeding of gorse and/or 3 to 4 lb. of raw potatoes daily will give relief, and to some extent arrest the development of the condition. Providing it is not in flower the gorse is cut, chaffed, and given mixed with oat straw, about two double hands full twice a day. One would think horses would not eat such prickly material but they appear to relish it.

Pneumonia The term Pneumonia is used to describe an inflammation of the lung tissues.

There are several forms of the disease named according to the part affected but for our purpose they can be considered as one.

The condition may result from exhaustion or exposure, due to these influences lowering the general resistance, thereby allowing germs which are normally present in the nose and lungs to become malignant. Medicines gaining access

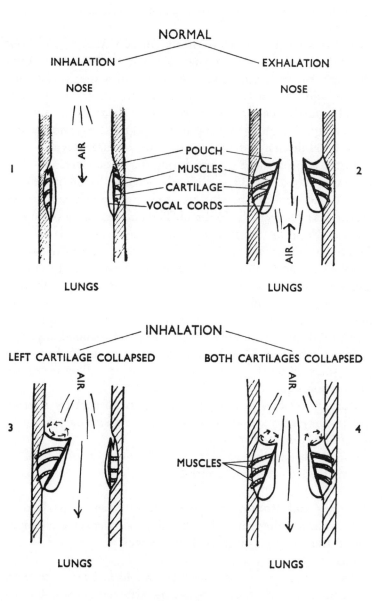

Fig. 33. Diagram of Larynx

to the lungs from careless drenching may set up pneumonia or it may follow some other disease such as Influenza or Strangles.

Symptoms The temperature rises from 105° to 107°, without any other development during the first twelve hours. After this lapse the breathing is increased, the pulse quick, shivering occurs and the ears, legs, and body are cold. The neck is usually outstretched, the nostrils dilated, and the stomach tucked up. Coughing occurs at the slightest exertion and a thick nasal discharge develops after two or three days.

Little improvement occurs during the critical period – five to seven days. Should the breath become foetid it usually means that serious changes are taking place in the lungs, in which case recovery is doubtful. The patient rarely lies down and the droppings are firm and often mucous coated.

Treatment Fresh air is absolutely essential. Warmth can be supplied in the form of rugs, bandages, hood, etc. but doors and windows should be left open, providing of course there is no draught. Inhalations of Eucalyptus of Friar's Balsam are beneficial. The diet is most important and should consist of green foods, linseed mashes, milk, eggs, and steamed hay.

If medicines are used they must be given in the form of a paste smeared on the tongue and teeth as drenching may have serious consequences.

Certain antibiotics are highly efficient, especially if given in the early stages, and in consequence *a Veterinary Surgeon should be consulted at once.*

In any event the patient must be given a long term of convalescence – several months.

Whistling and Roaring These conditions can be dealt with under one heading since the pathological changes are similar and differ only in degree. The changes are centred in the larynx.

The names explain themselves and have been coined to describe the noise that is made by affected horses, but its significance can be appreciated only if one has some

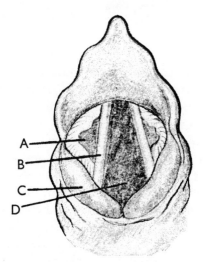

Fig. 34. Larynx of Horse: A. Opening into lateral ventricle in front of vocal fold; B. Vocal fold extending from the arytenoid cartilage to the epiglottis; C. Arytenoid cartilage; D. Rima glottidis or entrance into the trachea.

knowledge of the anatomy of the larynx.

This organ is a box-like structure whose walls are made up of cartilages united by joints and ligaments, lined on the inside by mucous membrane continuous with that of the throat and windpipe. The membrane is raised to form a pair of vocal folds each fold covering a ligament and a muscle. During inhalation the cartilages open, and at the same time draw the vocal cords with them, to allow of a free passage of air to the lungs. Both collapse on expiration.

The movement of the cartilages is controlled by three pairs of small muscles innervated by a slender nerve, one on either side, which pursue a somewhat tortuous route. They originate in the head and pass down the length of the neck in association with the carotid arteries on either side. At the base of the neck on the right side the nerve winds round a small artery and then runs up the jugular groove in the neck to the larynx. The left nerve passes back even further into the chest before it winds round the large main artery at the base of the heart and then follows the same course as the right nerve up the neck.

When dealing with nerve tissue earlier on I did not explain that their structure is such that should the outer covering or sheath become stretched, injured or inflamed, partial or complete destruction of the nerve will follow.

Sudden and excessive exertion such as galloping when at grass, or fast work too early in a horse's preparation will cause a sudden increase in blood flow and dilation of the blood vessels to accommodate such increase. This sudden dilation may not affect the right nerve as the variation in the small artery will not be appreciable. On the left side the nerve is much more vulnerable as the expansion of the large main artery is considerable and may easily cause stretching of the nerve resulting in its partial or complete destruction. Depending on the amount of damage to the nerve from any cause impulses to the small muscles become weaker as the nerve perishes and in consequence the movement of the cartilages will decrease. As the cartilages collapse so the vocal cords become slack and vibrate abnormally during inspiration. This vibration accounts for some of the whistle.

Another factor which contributes to this noise is the presence of a small pouch situated between the vocal cords and the cartilages. When the cartilages and vocal cords are slack this pouch is open and the inspired air passing over the mouth causes a whistle.

At first the noise may be slight and is called a whistle but as the collapse of the cartilage increases so the vibration of the slack cords becomes greater finally resulting in a much deeper sound known as roaring. A horse that whistles may well develop into a roarer but it is unusual for the reverse to occur, i.e. roarer to whistler.

A whistler or roarer is generally capable of easy work at slow paces but if exerted will show marked respiratory distress the sound becoming accentuated. During laboured respiration the laryngeal opening is normally widened to allow more air to flow in and out but in a whistler or roarer this increase cannot take place or at least only to a very small extent. The only reliable test for a horse's wind is therefore to make the horse perform some work and increase its breathing rate.

Other than the cause of whistling given above, which has some anatomical support, there are other theories, but none explain why the left side only is affected. As most Roarers and Whistlers have a history of some septic infection, such as strangles, damage to the nerves by toxins is a favourite idea. As the respiratory organs derive their nerve supply from the same source as does the stomach, diet and digestive upsets have been blamed.

There are other noises made by a horse during inspiration, which, to the unpractised ear, appear similar to the specific whistle, but which are not due to collapse of the cartilages, as in the case of:

a. Bridle noises. These are generally more muffled and occur when a horse is ridden in a severe bit, resulting in over flexion, which restricts the air passage in the larynx.

b. Over fat condition, causing inefficient movement of the cartilages.

c. Infections of the larynx, with only a slight cough, general in horses after a sea voyage. This may reduce the efficiency of the cartilages and cause a whistle until the initial trouble has resolved.

d. Infections of the glands and throat generally with visible symptoms of nasal discharge, enlarged glands, etc.

Finally, there are Intermittent Whistlers and Technical or False Whistlers.

In both cases, the typical whistle is heard but the condition in the larynx may never deteriorate.

The technical whistle, which is constant, might be the result of some permanent thickening of the larynx following an infection and although it may be so slight that it will not affect a horse's breathing, it must be judged to be an unsoundness as there is no certain method of discriminating between it and a true whistler.

To summarise, the existence of a typical whistle must be considered as the fore-runner of a progressive laryngeal paralysis, which could reduce the efficiency of any horse by as much as 75 per cent.

Treatment The only treatment is surgical, the operation consisting of removal of the membrane lining the laryngeal pouches.

As stated, in the sequence of healing of wounds, the cells formed between two cut edges have the power of contraction once the gap is bridged, bringing the edges together. In this operation, a surgical injury is occasioned by removal of the laryngeal pouches. The fibrous tissue which develops in the healing process contracts and the cord is pulled to the side of the larynx, leaving the lumen of that organ free from obstruction.

If performed when the condition is first noticed the operation gives a fair measure of success, but the chances of complete recovery are less as the condition progresses.

Preventive Measures It may not have occurred to some readers that whistling, other than in cases following strangles, or other throat infection, rarely develops during a season, but usually after a summer at grass. This fact adds support to the opinion that galloping when unfit, due to flies, etc., may cause damage to the nerves. Admittedly it is advantageous to turn a horse out to grass in the summer to give the system complete rest from concentrated food, but the writer is of the opinion that where one is the proud possessor of a valuable horse, yarding, or turning out in a very small paddock, with perhaps a donkey or very small pony, as a sobering influence, is preferable. In fact, in the case of a valuable heavy weight horse (so rare these days), because of the greater predisposition of this class to go wrong in the wind, the writer would not hesitate to keep the animal in the stable, and offer cut grass and occasional walking exercise during its rest period.

In the event of stabling, or yarding, being impractical,

galloping will be minimised by turning out by night and stabling by day.

Many experienced horsemen are of the opinion that conformation plays a part in this disease. Some say that long-necked horses are prone to this hazard. Others accuse the 'Bull Neck'. Such theories make interesting speculation.

Finally heredity is a major factor in the incidence of roaring and whistling, 'roarers beget roarers', hence breeding from affected horses should be avoided at all costs.

CHAPTER TWELVE

Skin Diseases

NON SPECIFIC

Warts, Warbles, Galls, Cracked Heels, Mud Fever, Grease,
Sweet Itch, Mallenders, Sallenders, Urticaria

Warts A wart is the name given to a tumour-like growth appearing on the skin. The shape may vary from cylindrical, with or without a neck, to flat or pointed.

The usual position for the cylindrical type is on the under surface of the stomach, on the sheath, between the hind legs, on the inner surface of the thigh, on the front of the chest and behind the point of the elbow.

The small pointed type are found usually on the nose, lips and ears.

Other tumour-like growths, which may be mistaken for warts, are pigment tumours and fibrous growths.

Pigment tumours, seen mostly in grey horses, appear usually at the side of the anus and below it, along the lower surface of the abdomen and inside the thighs. These tumours are formed underneath the skin and have no neck, the skin covering them being shiny.

Treatment Where a single wart with a well-defined stalk occurs, a fine piece of elastic tied round the neck will cut off the blood supply and the wart will die and drop off in time. This type is usually seen in numbers and then they require careful surgical removal.

In the case of the small pointed type, seen on the lips and nose, Col. Codrington found that a liberal supply of black treacle or engine sump oil applied daily for several days effected a cure in many cases! Caustics may be used, but most warts will recur if they are not removed carefully by an expert and in consequence *a Veterinary Surgeon should be consulted.*

Warbles Many flies have several stages in their life history as follows:

a. An adult fly lays eggs;

b. The eggs hatch out in the form of maggots, or larvae;

c. The maggot develops into an adult fly.

In the case of the warble fly, the female lands on the skin and lays her eggs during July, August and early September. The eggs hatch and the larvae find their way to the back and sides. During the winter nothing is seen, but in the early spring a hard nodule appears underneath the skin. Within a fortnight or so the swelling increases and eventually a small hole is seen in the summit of this swelling. Within a few days, providing the opening is large enough, slight pressure with the fingers will force the larva out, together with a little fluid, which may be blood-stained. The hole soon heals and the swelling subsides.

Treatment This must be directed towards hastening the eviction of the larva, and hot fomentations, or kaolin poultice, to soften the skin, will serve this purpose.

Providing the warble is not under the saddle or girth, no other treatment need be given. However, should pressure be applied, either by a saddle, or from squeezing before the larva is ready to appear, it will be killed with dire consequences. The infection following the bursting of the larva may cause a widespread swelling, which may persist for weeks and thereby incapacitate the animal for a long time.

From this it will be seen that any swelling of the skin occurring on the back or sides in the spring should be suspected as being due to a warble and, if under the saddle or girth, the animal should not be ridden until the cause has been established and, if a warble, until the larva has been expressed.

Kaolin poultices should not be used once a hole is seen, as they may stifle the larva, but hot fomentations applied instead.

In view of the danger of bursting the larva when trying to express it with the fingers, slight pressure only should be applied and if not successful, repeated on successive days.

Galls This term is employed to describe a soreness or laceration of the skin due to friction or undue pressure from saddlery. The areas affected are the skin immediately behind the point of the elbow on the ribs, known as girth galls, and the back underneath the seat of the saddle, known as sore backs or sit-fasts.

Girth Galls The main causes are:

a. Sensitive skin.

b. Too tight a girth when the animal is first ridden after a rest period.

c. Too loose a girth allowing excessive movement and consequent chafing.

d. Hard dirty girths which have become impregnated with stale sweat.

e. Sudden cooling of the skin when the girths are removed.

In some cases the bruising and consequent rupture of the small blood vessels may occur in the deeper layers of the skin resulting in a hard painful lump. In other cases the surface of the skin is affected, the hair being removed and the area raw.

Treatment The parts should be washed with warm salt water to remove any discharge, dried with swabs of cotton wool, and lightly dusted with sulphanilamide powder. The following day astringent lotions or a mild antiseptic ointment should be aplied.

If the area is small, about the size of a 50 penny piece, the girth may be doubled back to avoid further chafing and the animal ridden, but if a large area is affected complete healing must take place before the horse can be used again.

A great many girth galls can be prevented, even though the horse has a very sensitive skin. When first worked, after a rest period, a roller should be put on from the first day. The slight friction each time the animal moves will help to harden the skin gradually.

If the girths are made of webbing an inner motor tube or piece of sheepskin covering will minimise chafing but if well oiled rolled leather types are used covering is not necessary. Irrespective of the type all girths should be wiped over with a wet sponge after use, and hung up to dry, followed by a good brushing to remove all traces of sweat.

The object of loosening girths, but allowing the saddle to remain after returning to the stable, is to avoid sudden cooling of the skin which predisposes to galling.

Sore Back Galls occurring on the back are usually the result of pressure from a badly flocked saddle or from a tired rider who sits on the back of the saddle.

If the surface of the skin only is affected the same treatment as for girth galls will be adequate.

Another injury to the skin of this area is known as a **Sit-Fast**. In this condition a portion of skin dies owing to the circulation being completely cut off by pressure. The dead portion is cone shaped the base being uppermost. After a few days the dead portion separates from the living skin forming a fissure in which pus forms.

Treatment The dead portion must be removed before recovery can take place. Some advocate a mild blister around the base to bring more blood to the part and hasten separation, but kaolin poultices will have the same effect. The deep portion may not separate for some time and may require cutting out. After the 'core' has been removed the hole should be bathed twice daily with salt water to remove all discharge, followed by the application of penicillin ointment, and covered by a piece of cotton wool.

Even when the wound has healed a bare patch of skin will remain for some time, but further damage can be avoided by the use of a numnah with a hole cut over the area.

An ideal method to prevent sore backs is as follows. On returning to the stable remove the saddle and replace it by a numnah which has been kept warm by the fire or on hot pipes. Keep it in position with a roller and leave for at least an hour.

Cracked Heels This is an inflammatory condition of the skin of the heels, frequently caused by irritation from mud, or washing of the legs without drying them properly.

The skin becomes inflamed and the top layers die and collect as a sort of scurf. The hair stands up and the heels and fetlocks swell. The skin then becomes taut and eventually cracks, allowing infection to enter the deeper layers. Lameness occurs, the animal going on its toe to avoid bending the joint and stretching the skin. If the patient is made to move, on taking the first stride the pain, when flexing the heel, may be so acute that the leg is snatched up, sometimes so high that the animal loses its balance.

Treatment Dry heat applied in the form of hot boracic lint, as in the case of 'Mud Fever', is the most effective. At the same time, all concentrated foods should be withheld and a laxative, such as Epsom Salts (4 oz. in 1 pint of water) given. The diet should consist of soft hay and bran mashes until the inflammation has subsided and the cracks are healed.

To hasten healing, a daily application of acriflavine emulsion, or ichthammol ointment is useful. Exercise should be given when lameness ceases and it is advisable to bandage the legs for a time before going out, to avoid dirt and moisture aggravating the condition. On returning to the stable, the bandages should be removed, the legs massaged lightly, and after a few hours, rebandaged. This assists circulation and promotes healing.

Prevention As in the case of 'Mud Fever', if the legs are very dirty, they should not be washed or cleaned the same night, but cotton wool and bandages applied and left until the following morning.

If it is known that a horse is susceptible to skin irritation, a heavy oil, such as castor oil, applied to the heels before hunting may prevent the condition.

Mud Fever This is a condition in which the skin becomes inflamed as a result of irritation often from mud, hence the name.

The usual site of the trouble is in the lower part of the limbs from the knee and hock downward, but the under surface of the belly may also be affected.

Horses are particularly susceptible to this ailment because the percentage of blood circulating in the skin is much higher than in other animals. In consequence the skin is more prone to congestion.

Although the condition may occur in horses at grass in a very wet season the type we are concerned with here applies to corn fed animals in the stable.

Certain soils are more irritant to the skin than others, especially those containing silicates. These are minute pointed crystals, which can penetrate the skin and having done so can travel about in the underlying tissue. The small breaches in the skin allow infective germs to enter.

Symptoms In the first instance the legs become swollen and hot. As the swelling increases, circulation is hindered, the blood vessels become congested, serum oozes out of them and collects on the skin. Owing to the blood supply being impaired the top layers of the skin die, cracks may form and infection will gain access through these fissures. The hair stands erect and the patient moves with a stiff gait.

Treatment Before dealing with any method of treatment one should bear in mind the great part played by the skin in elimination. If the animal is having a quantity of corn it should be reduced or discontinued at once, in order to avoid further irritation from that source. A mild purgative may be given to increase elimination from the bowel and so relieve the skin of some of its work.

Dry heat should be applied to dilate the blood vessels and so reduce congestion. The most effective method of applying dry heat is by means of boracic lint. A piece the length and circumference of the leg is rolled up and placed on a clean stable rubber which has been spread over a tin or other flat receptacle. *Boiling* water is poured on the lint, the stable rubber is picked up by the corners and twisted in opposite directions until all the water has been squeezed out of the lint. *As quickly as possible* the lint is wrapped around the leg, covered by a liberal wrapping of cotton wool, and bandaged immediately. This process should be repeated twice daily. Although two people are required to implement the treatment, seeing that speed is the all-important factor, results will warrant the extra trouble.

Once the lint has cleansed the skin of all discharge and the inflammation is subsiding, cooling lotions may be used and the animal sent to exercise. At first movement will reduce the swelling, but it will return when at rest. As work is increased the filling will gradually subside.

In the event of sore areas persisting after the lint treatment, cooling lotions should be avoided and an antiseptic ointment applied to the areas. An ointment containing Ichthyol is very efficient in these cases.

Bandages should be worn in the stable for some time to keep the parts at a regular warm temperature and to assist circulation.

Prevention Because mud fever is so often due to faulty management, prevention is all-important and should be the main safe-guard. Certain soils are worse than others, but if the correct stable routine is adopted, the type of mud is immaterial.

We know that when a horse returns from a 'hard day' the system will be in a state of fatigue and as the skin is controlled by the nervous system, the pores of the skin will be relaxed. In an effort to make the animal comfortable, one would expect to clean the limbs with a brush or straw wisp, but this is a very foolish practice. By so doing the irritant mud will be forced into the open pores of the skin, and when the animal regains normal tone after rest, the pores will close and imprison the mud particles. All soil contains germs which are capable of infecting living tissue and the tissues respond by becoming irritated and inflamed.

If cotton wool and bandages are applied, to conserve body heat, and the legs are left to dry off before grooming, the pores close normally and scarcely, if ever, will mud fever occur.

Grease is a chronic inflammation of the skin, usually of the hind legs below the hock, but occasionally the fore legs may be affected. Heavy horses, especially those with a lot of hair, are prone to the condition, but it is seldom seen in the lighter types. The cause is unknown although it is considered by some to be due to excessive protein in the food, but it may appear out at grass so that this can only be an influence and not the cause of the condition. Bacterial invasion of the inflammatory areas generally occurs.

Symptoms The skin becomes swollen and inflamed. Later there is a discharge, which collects on the surface of the skin and has a very offensive odour. The leg is wet with this discharge and the hair stands on end. The leg may swell and the skin become very thickened.

Treatment should be active and immediate. Clipping affected areas and washing with mild soap followed by the application of a mild astringent. If treatment is delayed, it may be very difficult to effect a cure, and in consequence *a Veterinary Surgeon should be consulted.*

Sweet Itch This is a skin condition seen mostly in small ponies, but other types may be affected.

It is of seasonal occurrence, being prevalent in spring and summer, and is seen only in animals at grass or fed green food in the stable.

Symptoms Areas of skin on the mane, neck, tail and withers become inflamed and very sensitive and in consequence, the animal rubs itself against any object. The upper layers of the skin become damaged and serum is exuded and collects on the surface as a yellowish deposit. The hair falls out, leaving moist bare patches.

Treatment As the condition may be an allergic response to some component in grass, if practicable green foods should be avoided. In many cases this is not possible. Affected areas should be clipped and cleansed with water containing a trace of washing soda. After washing the area can be treated with calomine lotion or a weak astringent lotion of alum. Should

the condition persist and exhibit pus formation sulphanilamide powder may be considered. It can also be kept under
control by a weekly dressing with Kur-Mange obtained from
any chemist. The contents of one tin are dissolved in one
quart of warm water and this is brushed gently into the
affected areas and allowed to dry on the skin. Benzyl
benzoate applied every other day is useful. Sun's rays are
claimed to aggravate the condition, the animal being turned
out at night only. Finally, antihistamines may be tried, but in
all cases of eczema it is advisable to consult a veterinary
surgeon since the possibility of the condition being the result
of parasitic mange must be eliminated.

Mallenders and Sallenders These are names given to an
inflammation of the skin occurring at the back of the knee
and in front of the hock respectively.

Following on the inflammation, dead flakes of skin collect,
the patches being dry and dark grey. As these lesions are sited
in the bends of the joints the skin often cracks and becomes
ulcerated. Lameness may occur.

Treatment The condition can be very obstinate to cure,
especially if treatment be delayed. The scales and any
discharge can be removed by a good washing with hot water
and toilet soap, to which a little bicarbonate of soda has been
added. This should be followed by the application of an
antiseptic ointment, well massaged into the part daily.
Iodine, salicylic acid, or ichthammol ointments are all useful.
It is wise to alternate the dressings as the condition will
respond to one of them in one animal and not in another.
Even in the case of one animal it is a good practice to change
the dressing from time to time.

Urticaria This is a condition of the skin and it is considered
to be an allergic reaction to some component of the diet.

Areas varying in size from a penny to the palm of one's
hand, or larger, become raised and the hair on the patches is
erect. They develop suddenly and may disappear in a very

short time. Unlike the condition in humans there is no irritation and the appearance of the skin is normal.

The condition may occur where corn and hard hay is not cut down during a short period of rest, or as a sequel to strangles.

Treatment In horses treatment is rarely necessary, as the lesions disappear as rapidly as they arrive. However, if corn or hard hay has not been reduced during the rest period, this should be done and a laxative such as Epsom Salts be given in the water. A cooling lotion can be applied such as Calomine or the affected areas may be treated with a strong solution of bicarbonate of soda in water — two tablespoonsful to the pint. The solution should be applied liberally. Injection of either of the anti-histamine group or cortisone will often hasten recovery. Antibiotics may also be useful to prevent infection from occurring.

SPECIFIC SKIN DISEASES
Mange, Ringworm, Heel Bug

Mange There are three types of mange which affect horses, viz.: Sarcoptic, Psoroptic and Symbiotic. Each is highly contagious and is caused by a parasite.

Sarcoptic Mange This parasite affects mostly the withers, back, neck, shoulders and sides. Small lumps appear on the skin and a yellowish liquid oozes from them, which dries, the hair falls out and a dry scaly patch is left. There is intense irritation of the skin, especially when the animal is warm, and it is constantly rubbing and biting itself. If the areas are scratched the horse will extend its neck and make characteristic nibbling movements with its lower lip.

Psoroptic Mange is similar to the former but is less irritant and usually is found at the base of the mane and tail.

The only sure method of differentiating between these two forms is by microscopic examination of the parasite.

Both types of mange are scheduled diseases and suspected cases must be notified to the police. The Ministry of Agriculture then comes on the scene. If the outbreak is confirmed control and treatment are under the supervision of a Veterinary Officer of the Animal Health Division.

Symbiotic Mange is a comparatively benign condition affecting the legs from the knee and hock downwards. It is characterised by irritation, stamping and attempts to bite and rub the legs. The skin becomes thickened and scaly and the hair falls out of the affected parts.

Treatment consists of clipping the hair and washing the legs thoroughly twice weekly for three weeks, followed by the application of an anti-parasite dressing containing Derris Root. Benzene hydrochloride and the organophosphorus compounds such as Diazinon are effective mite killers but *the prescription for their use must be left to the veterinary surgeon.*

Ringworm This is a contagious disease caused by a fungus. Circular areas of hair become raised, a small amount of fluid exudes from the skin and the hair becomes matted and falls out, leaving a bald patch covered with dry greyish scales. These areas extend outward, but usually retain their circular shape.

As the fungus lives under the scales, these must be removed by scrubbing or scraping the areas before any medicament is applied. Iodine, in the form of an ointment, is the usual treatment, but painting with an aniline dye, called Gentian Violet, is equally efficient. A dichlorophen spray is also a convenient method of application of treatment. Dressings should be carried out twice a week for a fortnight. Recently periodic administration orally of the antibiotic griseofulvin for several weeks has proved successful.

Difficulty may arise in determining when the condition is cured, but generally speaking, when no further scales form and the hair begins to grow one can be reasonably certain that the lesion is cured.

Ringworm is a highly contagious disease and strict hygienic measures must be adopted to prevent its spreading to other areas on the affected animal and to other horses. The affected animal should be isolated. Grooming kit, harness, and clothing should be washed and disinfected frequently. Walls, mangers, stable equipment, etc., should be treated in like manner. It is best to burn bedding.

Heel Bug The name Heel Bug has been given to an infection of the skin affecting the heels and lower limbs of horses, but the causal agent is not known.

The infection is highly contagious. It is observed most frequently in race horses in training.

Symptoms Slight swelling. Local inflammatory reaction in the skin and a stiffness in action are the first signs to be noticed. Within six hours swelling in the heels has increased considerably and the legs begin to swell. The skin is very taut and shiny, the hair stands on end and a thick yellow discharge oozes from the glands in the skin of the heel.

At first one might consider the condition a mud fever, but the rate at which the heels swell and the tenseness of the skin are diagnostic. In a white leg the skin soon becomes blue tinged.

Treatment Hot dry lint applied as in Mud Fever is useful. A similar type of treatment is with plain flour. A stocking is pulled over the leg, bandaged at the hoof and flour poured in and lightly bandaged at the top. The application should be changed every six hours.

The use of Antiphlogistine or any ointment should be avoided as the condition will be aggravated. Laxatives, mashes and a hay diet should be given.

Owing to the highly infectious nature of the condition, every precaution must be taken in disinfecting bedding, grooming utensils, etc.

Because the condition occurs generally in race horses in spring and summer time, there is a suggestion that the infection may be picked up in the dewy grass and that the thin skin of a thoroughbred is more susceptible than that of coarser bred animals.

It has been suggested also that the infecting agent gains access through minute punctures in the skin, occasioned by the sharp edges and points of the grass. Others think that there may be some irritant substance in the dew or in the juices expressed when the grass is bruised by the horse's feet. The infective theory is supported by the fact that the condition will extend to other animals which have been clear previously, if an affected horse be admitted to the stable.

CHAPTER THIRTEEN

Diseases of Circulation

Heart Disease Heart diseases can only be properly recognized by the highly trained, professional observer although many owners may suspect their presence. Their treatment and an estimation of the effect they will have in the long term on the life of the horse must be entrusted to a Veterinary Surgeon. With these preliminary warning words in mind we can just mention one or two things about the action of the heart generally. As described in the section on the circulation of the blood the return flow to the heart passes into the two atria, right and left, and when both are full the walls contract to force the blood into the right and left ventricles. Between each atrium and its corresponding ventricle there is an opening guarded by a flap valve. When open this valve permits the blood to flow from atrium to ventricle since at this time the ventricle is relaxed. Once the ventricle is full with incoming blood the valve closes with an audible sound (i.e. if one's ear or a stethoscope is placed over the heart area of the chest wall) and the ventricular muscle contracts to force the blood either to the lungs or the body. Between each ventricle and the large vessels leading from them there are valves; a pulmonary valve in the artery leading to the lungs and an aortic valve in the artery conveying blood to the body generally. At the end of ventricular contraction when the ventricles have emptied of blood the walls relax and these two valves close with another audible sound. Two basic sounds can therefore be heard in one heart cycle and they differ in tone. The sounds are best described by the words LUBB – DUP. The longer, deeper LUBB sound is related to the atrioventricular valves; DUP is a short sound corresponding to the closure of the pulmonary and aortic valves.

Any deviation from this normal sequence of LUBB – DUP may be considered as heart disease. Similarly when a beat is missed it is known as an Intermittence and this should be considered as abnormal. However there are two types of intermittence known as Regular and Irregular.

A Regular Intermittence is not serious and may be due to lack of condition, indigestion, etc. It may be present when the animal is resting in the stable but disappears on exercise.

An Irregular Intermittence can be much more serious and is usually due to valve failure.

Because any intermittence or unusual sound, following or preceding Lubb or Dup, may be serious, it is essential that a Veterinary Surgeon be called at once.

Other than murmurs caused by inefficiency of the valves, any irregularity can be accounted for quite accurately by submitting the animal to an electro-cardiograph. This machine can settle many differences of opinion with a high degree of accuracy.

Epistaxis This is the term used to describe bleeding from the nose. The cause is not known. It often happens after excessive exertion and occurs in both fit and unfit horses. It has been known to occur when the animal was at rest. Col. Codrington recorded that on two occasions several horses in one training stable were affected during a period of six to seven weeks.

The membranes of the nose are very delicate and richly supplied with blood. It is conceivable that any influence which causes a sudden increased blood flow, such as violent or prolonged exertion, or even inflammation from dusty fodder, might bring about a rupture of the thin-walled blood vessels. However, when bleeding originates in the nostrils themselves there is never much blood loss and the animal may have repeated attacks without any serious consequences.

Lack of calcium in the blood, resulting in loss of tone of the blood vessels, has been suggested as a possible cause.

Bleeding from one nostril is commonly of nasal origin.

Epistaxis can also occur as a secondary manifestation of some other respiratory condition when bleeding will probably occur from both nostrils. In recent years a condition described as diphtheria of the guttural pouch has been suggested as being the major cause of nose bleeding. This pouch leads off from the throat and its mucous membrane lining is attacked by diphtheritic organisms. Damaged blood vessels may discharge spontaneously while the horse is at rest into the pouch from where it flows into the pharynx or down the nose. Since diphtheria is a readily transmissible disease it may account for the observation made on the previous page by Col. Codrington that several horses in one training stable were affected during a six or seven week period.

Treatment Should the condition occur during a race, the bleeding usually stops soon after the horse has pulled up, but if it persists, the affected nostril can be plugged.

Complete rest and a laxative diet should be given.

The safest plan is to throw the horse out of training for the season, but even this will not ensure a cure, especially in a horse over eight years old.

Epistaxis due to guttural pouch diphtheria has so little known about the specific organism causing it that any line of treatment would be purely speculative. The pouch may be irrigated and antibiotic injections utilized.

Filled Legs In the chapter on circulation it was explained that lack of exercise would lead to a poor circulation, especially in the limbs. If too much concentrated food is given the waste products are not eliminated as quickly and efficiently as they should be and the lymphatic vessels and the tissue become congested.

Any debilitating condition, especially one affecting the bowel, may cause this type of congestion and filled legs are one of the visible manifestations.

A simple case of filled legs may be seen in a horse that is brought in from grass and fed corn before the system has been prepared to deal with the new diet. A laxative diet should be given for the first few days, followed by a mild purgative. After the purgative, give hay and a daily mash for a few days and then commence with a small quantity of corn.

The time of preparation for work can be shortened considerably by giving two to three pounds of corn daily for a month before bringing the horse in. If this is done a purgative is not necessary. A few days of a laxative diet will be sufficient before giving normal dry feeds.

Some horses are subject to filled legs. The commoner type of hunter seems to be most subject to this hazard, due no doubt to the fact that they are unable to deal as adequately with a large corn ration as is a thoroughbred.

A filled leg will often occur in a limb that has been injured. When an animal has sustained an appreciable injury, damage to some of the blood vessels is certain to occur and the circulation is impaired. A sluggish circulation can be stimulated and improved by the use of bandages, hand-rubbing, massage, and regular exercise.

Lymphangitis When dealing with the circulation, it was explained that blood was carried by the arteries to all parts of the body and was returned to the heart by the veins. A similar system of vessels, called the lymphatics, also carries waste products from all parts of the body back to the heart. At intervals along these pipes there are masses of tissue, called lymphatic glands, or nodes, whose function is to 'hold up' any infection present in the lymph fluid and so prevent the germs from gaining access to the blood stream. The most obvious examples of this function are to be seen in the head and throat. Infections of the throat, as in coughs and colds, are usually evidenced by swelling of the lymphatic glands in this area.

The term Lymphangitis, or inflammation of the lymphatic vessels, is applied to a condition occurring usually in the hind limbs of horses as a result of excessive corn diet, coupled with lack of work. It often appears in horses after coming in from a time at grass and put straight on to hard corn feeding.

This emphasises the importance of following the preparation sequence of a horse as set out in chapter 16.

Symptoms Unlike ordinary 'filled legs', the swelling is much greater and stops suddenly at the level of the stifle, forming a diagnostic 'ridge' around the limb. The actual lymphatic vessels on the inside of the thigh become so enlarged that they are easily visible, and slight pressure on them will cause considerable pain.

The temperature may rise to 105°, sweating and blowing are evident, and the animal shows great distress. Lameness is acute.

Treatment A mild purgative may be given to assist the elimination of waste products, followed by a laxative diet. Hot fomentations with a large blanket applied to the thigh region, will assist the circulation.

A free supply of water should be offered. To each bucket of water should be added a tablespoon of epsom salts and one small teaspoon of potassium nitrate, the former to assist elimination by the bowel and the latter to stimulate the kidneys. Gentle massage of the affected limb, with or without a mild embrocation, can be performed in an upward direction.

Once the swelling has begun to subside, light exercise should be given but corn should not be given until the animal is fit to work again. It is best to stop feeding oats, beans or peas when the animal is not working, as the condition will often recur after the first attack. Usually the affected limb remains slightly thicker after the first attack and this permanent enlargement increases with each successive attack. It is wise to give a horse that has suffered one attack half an hours walking or lungeing during a rest day or to turn it out into a paddock for a while.

Azoturia Known also as Myohaemoglobinuria, is a condition occurring in corn fed animals when the corn has not been reduced during a rest period, such as is occasioned by frost, etc.

The actual cause has not been determined.

Symptoms Any time from ten to thirty minutes after leaving the stable, especially if the horse is at all fresh, the stride behind is shortened, followed soon by a distinct stiffness of the loins. Profuse sweating and blowing occur and if the animal is allowed to stand for a few minutes, on moving there is great distress. Soon after the onset of symptoms groups of muscles on the loins and quarters become very hard and painful to the touch. When urine is passed it is seen to be coffee coloured and there is a distinct smell of violets. The coloured urine and hardened quarter muscles are absolutely diagnostic. The temperature may rise 2°−3°.

Treatment In mild attacks the animal should be kept walking to get him back to the stable, but if the attack is acute a box must be sent for.

On return to the stable hot blankets should be applied to the loins *and professional advice sought at once,* as timely treatment will often effect a quick cure.

Where an attack has occurred there would appear to be a susceptibility to recurrence, in which case care must be taken to stop all corn and offer a laxative diet should the horse be rested for any reason. Further, even during regular work, it is advisable to give the animal a short canter daily.

CHAPTER FOURTEEN

Diseases of the Eye

Because of the delicate nature of the tissues of the eye, and the serious results that can follow lack of early treatment by an expert, only the simple conditions will be considered.

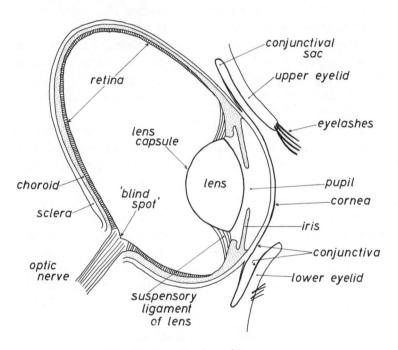

Fig. 35. Cross Section of Eye

Injury Bruising of the eyelids and the bones forming the eye socket may result from a blow. The eyelids become swollen and there is an excessive formation of tears. If the eyeball shows no change the case can be considered as a simple injury and will respond to ordinary fomentation.

If the lids are torn every effort should be made to preserve all of the fragments and veterinary assistance should be obtained immediately in order to stitch them. Normally the upper and lower lids fit perfectly, and by their constant movement cleanse the eyeball of dirt and infection. If a torn lid is not stitched a gap will result allowing infection and dust to collect in the eye.

Conjunctivitis This is the term used to denote an inflammation of the membrane covering the inside of the eyelids, known as the conjunctiva. It may result from injury, irritation from dust or other irritant material, or the presence of a foreign object, or it may be a complication of a systemic disease, e.g. Strangles. Generally it is not in itself a serious condition but it may produce complications such as keratitis (see below).

Symptoms The membrane becomes deep red, the eyelids are swollen, there is an excessive flow of tears and usually a sticky mucous discharge forms which runs down the face from the inner corner. This discharge may blister the facial skin over which it trickles.

Treatment Any irritant body present should be removed at once and the eye irrigated with warm water. If the case is a simple inflammation following a blow, flushing of the eye with a solution of epsom salts several times a day for a few days should effect a cure. The correct strength of the solution is 1 teaspoon of epsom salts to 1 pint of boiled water.

Incidentally all water used to bathe eyes should have been boiled before use. Most waters contain salts which are irritant to the eye but they are deposited by boiling.

Should infection follow conjunctivitis, as evidenced by a discharge, the treatment will need to be more severe. Flushing is necessary to remove the excess of discharge after which one of the antibiotics in ointment form should be used. Ointment is preferable to a watery solution of an antiseptic, as the latter, even if used at full strength, will be diluted by the tears and thus reduce its efficiency.

If the conjunctivitis is a complication of some general disease treatment will be included in the latter.

Keratitis This is the term used to describe an inflammation of the membrane forming the front of the eyeball, known as the cornea. It may result from a direct injury, from infection of the conjunctiva, or from a foreign object.

Symptoms Unlike other tissue which becomes red when inflamed, the cornea becomes bluey white (comparable to the changes which take place in the white of an egg when heated). This is due to the fact that the cornea is not nourished by blood flowing in blood vessels since this would reduce the amount of light entering the eye. Instead, it possesses large numbers of spaces between the cells in which lymph circulates. It is the clotting of lymph which leads to corneal opacity. Early symptoms of the condition will be similar to those for conjunctivitis. The area affected will depend on the extent of the injury or infection. Occasionally a small hole, known as an ulcer, may be seen on the surface and is a serious complication as it is often difficult to heal and will leave a permanent scar. A mild keratitis may result from an animal rubbing a blistered leg with its head, some of the blister getting into the eye. Although alarming to see, usually the inflammation soon settles down without treatment.

Another frequent cause of this condition is the presence of an oat husk. Being almost transparent it may not be noticed at first as it lies flat on the cornea, the only symptom being excessive tears. If not removed the area around the husk becomes opaque after two or three days, and the actual husk can be seen as a yellow area.

Treatment A simple inflammation will usually respond to flushing the eye with epsom salts solution followed by some antibiotic ointment, as in the case of conjunctivitis. However if an oat husk is present it must be removed immediately otherwise serious damage will follow. Similarly if a wound or ulcer exists expert advice must be called.

Cataract For general purposes cataract is the only condition that need be considered under anatomical changes. To appreciate the actual state reference should be made to the diagram of the eye. It will be seen that the lens is an egg-shaped structure made up of concentric layers of material much like the leaves of an onion the whole surrounded by an outer membrane. This membrane may crease or even rupture as the result of a blow or infection, the nutrition of the lens is interrupted and the plasma of the lens cells coagulates causing a blurred vision, as would occur if one of the lenses in a pair of binoculars was shattered. Often a cataract is a progressive condition, and although sight may not be affected much in the initial stages, total blindness may be the final outcome. This fact makes it imperative that an expert opinion be sought when buying a horse as the cursory examination of an eye will not reveal the presence pf a cataract in the early stages.

Several methods have been suggested to reveal a cataract but, with the exception of an Ophthalmoscope in the hands of an expert, none are reliable.

One such method was the employment of a lighted candle which was passed backwards and forwards in front of the eye. If the eye is normal three reflections of the flame should be seen — one from the cornea, one from the front surface of the lens, and the third from the back surface of the lens. If either of the latter two is absent or indistinct it might signify some changes taking place in the fluid of the lens. In any case it is not at all accurate, especially in the early stages, as creasing of the membrane, often the forerunner of a rupture, will not affect the images.

Treatment There is no cure as the damaged tissue cannot be replaced.

Blindness may be caused by many things, it may be congenital or acquired, temporary or permanent, partial or complete. If it is only partial or affecting one eye, it may not be easy to detect at once. Three methods which may give one some indication of defective sight are as follows:

The rough test is to thrust a finger at the ball of the eye, the assumption being that if the animal is blind it will not blink the eyelids. This test is by no means infallible as the slight movement of air caused by the sudden movement of the hand may be felt by the animal and result in a blink.

Walk the animal across a yard, then place a large log or object about a foot high on the ground, cover one eye with a rubber and walk him back over the object. If he can see he will look down at the object and then lift his leg over it. Repeat with the other eye closed. If he cannot see he will walk into the object.

Stand the animal in a strong light and with the fingers open and close the eyelids. If the pupil becomes smaller when the eyelids are opened it indicates that the nerve supply to the eye is not affected.

CHAPTER FIFTEEN

Specific Diseases

Strangles This is the name given to a contagious disease peculiar to the horse tribe, the main evidence of which is abscess formation in the glands situated behind and underneath the lower jaw bone. Usually it attacks the young animal, but in a serious outbreak in a stable, horses of all ages may be affected. It is not often that an animal gets a second attack.

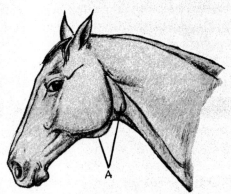

Fig. 36. Strangles
A. Glands Affected

Predisposing causes apart from age are numerous, such factors as overcrowding, bad ventilation, overexcitement, overwork of young horses, and the season of the year, will all affect the incidence of the condition. The causal agent itself is bacterial.

The seriousness of the disease lies in the fact that the animal is out of work for several weeks and there is always the possibility of permanent damage to the throat, resulting in whistling or roaring.

Symptoms Loss of appetite, dullness, rise of 2° to 3° temperature and enlarged glands in the region of the head. Usually the first glands to be affected are those underneath the jaw and often the type of swelling is diagnostic. Whereas the swollen gland seen in this area in an ordinary cold is soft and bilateral, a strangles abscess is hot, tense, painful and frequently one side only is affected. *Further, this abscess appears to be adherent to the inner surface of the jaw.*

Occasionally the glands between the jaw and the ear are also enlarged. The gland under the jaw is hard at first, but after a few days, it becomes soft and bursts and heals within a few days.

A thick yellow discharge from the nose occurs, accompanied by a cough.

Treatment Owing the the highly contagious nature of the disease, great care must be taken to isolate the animal and disinfect all utensils and tools frequently.

The horse should be put in a well-ventilated box and rugs and bandages applied.

Soft foods and mashes should be given and fomentations applied to the abscess to hasten its ripening and bursting. Occasionally, the abscess is slow in coming to a head, in which case a very light application of a mild blister may hasten the process. The object in inducing the abscess to burst is to avoid the infection spreading to the rest of the body. Should this happen, serious consequences may follow, recovery is quicker once the abscess has matured and discharged its contents.

Penicillin injections are generally of great value in reducing the severity of the attack and speeding recovery, while sulpha drugs have also provided useful. A suitable vaccine has lately been produced and gives a serviceable immunity although untoward reactions may occur.

Electuaries to soothe the inflamed throat will help the animal to feed.

Since complications may readily arise due to the spread of

pus and infective organisms in the blood stream to other parts of the body a veterinary surgeon must be called in.

Debility and loss of condition may follow an attack of strangles and it is therefore a wise plan to give the animal a long rest after an attack — at least six weeks. Good nourishing food is most important at this time. The horse whose period of convalescence occurs in the months of April and June, is lucky, for 'Dr Green' in the fresh young grass is the best Doctor of all.

Tetanus is a specific disease caused by a germ gaining access to the body by means of a wound. It lives normally in the soil in the form of a spore and can remain as such for years.

On entering the body the protective covering dissolves and the germ starts to propagate. During growth the germ produces a toxic material which affects the nervous system, the symptoms varying with the group or groups of muscles concerned. The period between the entry into the body and the onset of symptoms will vary from five to twenty days, or even longer.

Symptoms These vary considerably according to the virulence of the disease, but in some form or another, stiffness will be noticed at the outset. Feeding is slow and breathing is quicker.

At this juncture, or even before any symptom beyond slight stiffness is noticed, examination of the eye will give you a very early clue. If the hand is put under the lower jaw and the head raised, a small membrane, commonly called the 'Haw', in the corner of the eye will be seen to protrude and may even cover three parts of the front of the eyeball.

To effect a cure early treatment is essential and as this eye symptom is one of the first *typical* clinical signs to be observed, its importance should be appreciated.

As the disease progresses further symptoms are evidenced; viz. sweating, difficulty in eating or even swallowing, in which case frothing occurs, due to the collection of saliva and inability to swallow it. The tail is held high and quivers,

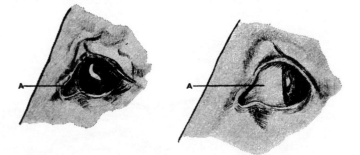

Fig. 37. Tetanus
left   Normal eye with nictitating membrane (Haw) labelled A in
the inner angle of the eye
right Eye in tetanus showing membrane partly covering eyeball (A)

nostrils are dilated, and the lips are drawn and teeth exposed. Generally speaking the more rapid the onset of symptoms, the more likely is the case to prove fatal. Should the patient get down the case is hopeless.

Treatment Because the germ remains in and around the wound, the symptoms being caused by their toxin getting into the blood, where practicable the wound should be enlarged and a strong antiseptic applied.

Until recently Tetanus Anti-serum was the only treatment available, and in some cases it had a beneficial effect, but a number of cases did not respond, partly due to the fact that an allergic reaction to the serum developed which aggravated the disease. It is now known that the germ is sensitive to penicillin with streptomycin. Provided the case is diagnosed early a single large dose of anti-serum is given immediately, followed the next day with a large dose of penicilln with streptomycin, and continued daily until the nervous symptoms abate — generally after five to six days. By this method many cases will be cured. Bran mashes with laxatives should be given, or where the jaws are immovable liquid diet such as milk and eggs. If the weather is good, and an isolated

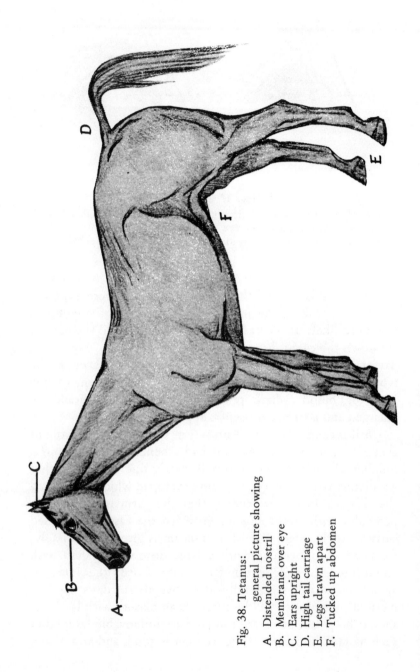

Fig. 38. Tetanus:
　general picture showing
A. Distended nostril
B. Membrane over eye
C. Ears upright
D. High tail carriage
E. Legs drawn apart
F. Tucked up abdomen

field without ditches or ponds is available, it is preferable to keep the patient out to avoid unnecessary stiffness.

Even if a cure is effected a long rest is essential.

With regard to prevention it was usual to give a dose of serum at the time of an injury, but cases can occur from wounds which are never discovered. In any event this type of immunity was only effective for about three to four weeks. A type of vaccine is now available which will produce a permanent immunity. The initial dose is given followed by a second dose one month later, and a final dose one year later. *If only on economical grounds this immunisation is advisable, and a certificate obtained from the Veterinary Surgeon at the time so that it can be given to a purchaser in the event of a sale.* If there is no evidence that an animal has been vaccinated when purchased, even though it may have been, a second course would have no ill effect.

Fistulous Withers This is a condition in which an abscess occurs at the point and side of the withers. In this region the supraspinous bursa lies over the thoracic spines between these and the nuchal ligament. The bursa is under considerable tension because of this overlying tissue, and therefore bursal inflammation is particularly serious. Because of the prominence of the withers this area is vulnerable to injury and it has been suggested that an infection centres in the bursa and/or the damaged muscles following such injury. Further, because the muscles are in layers, an infection can run rife with little chance of effective drainage.

Causes Pinches from saddlery;

Injury from blows when entering very low sheds;

Injury from rolling on hard ground;

Damage to tissue by bites from another horse.

Following injury from any of these causes the type of infection which may result may be either:

a. Any of the pus-producing organisms;

b. The same germ that causes abortion in cattle.

Symptoms There are certain symptoms which are sufficiently diagnostic to help in deciding which type of infection one is dealing with.

Infection from pus-producing organisms	*Infection from the Abortion Bacillus*
1. The initial swelling appears on the top and just below the point of the withers.	The initial swelling tends to appear on the side of the withers.
2. There is intense inflammation on both sides of the withers.	The inflammation is not so acute.
3. The area of the point of the abscess is large and the surrounding skin hard.	The area is smaller and a fluid abscess occurs.
4. When the abscess breaks, the material is a thick yellow discharge.	The contents of the abscess are fluid and may contain little or no pus.
5. Abscess formation is accompanied by considerable pain.	Pain is much less.
6. A laboratory test of blood is negative.	A laboratory test is positive.

It has been said that either type is contagious, but it is quite possible that should more than one case occur there may be common cause of injury, such as ill- fitting collars or saddles.

Treatment Because the layers of muscles prevent a proper drainage, the condition is difficult to cure and requires a major operation in the case of an infection from the pus-producing germs.

In the event of the condition being caused by the Abortion Bacillus, besides surgical interference, a series of injections with Abortion Vaccine may help to effect a cure.

It is well to remember that the discharge from such a case is highly infectious and great care must be taken to isolate the animal and disinfect all bedding and drains to avoid spread.

The incidence of Fistulous Withers is not so great as was the case some years ago. As most of the cases are due to injury the more precise attention that is paid to the fitting of harness and saddlery today may be paying a welcome dividend.

Poll Evil This is an infection of the tissues in the region of the Atlas, the first neck bone, and affecting the bursa interposed between the latter bone and the main ligament of the neck which runs from the withers to the base of the skull. Usually it occurs as a result of a blow or ill-fitting bridle with infection following in the damaged tissue

Symptoms A swelling occurs on either side of the middle line of the neck immediately behind the ears. As in the case of fistulous withers an abscess forms and there is swelling and pain.

Treatment is surgical and the sooner the surgeon can get to work the better are the prospects of a cure.

PART III

MANAGEMENT

CHAPTER SIXTEEN

Stable Management

When attending any animal all efforts should be directed towards the maintenance of health and prevention of disease, and as the latter is as much a Veterinary matter as cure I have included this chapter.

It has been said that too close a comparison is made between the training of animals and humans, but a notable exception to this is the case of an extremely successful National Hunt trainer, whose early life was, I understand, devoted entirely to the training of athletes.

To a great extent the secret of success in animal management can be summed up in the old saying. 'The eye of the Master maketh the horse'. Animals vary a great deal in character, and individuals may change from day to day, and unless one is watching constantly such variations will not be noticed and appropriate treatment applied. I refer to the Shy Feeder, the Night Feeder, the horse that bolts his food, etc.

Before going into details there are two main features peculiar to the horse which govern a successful approach to their management.

1. The stomach is small in comparison to the size of the gut. Food, after being masticated by the teeth, passes down into the stomach where it remains for at least an hour to allow the digestive juices to act on it and prepare it for the final digestion in the gut. Large feeds, especially if eaten quickly, may overload the stomach and a portion of the food will pass into the gut before due preparation, resulting in malnutrition.
2. The stomach and gut are particularly sensitive and in consequence react adversely to any sudden change. Enough of generalisation and let us commence with a

horse that has just come up off grass and is required for work. Whether the animal is intended for hacking, hunting or racing the method of training will vary only in detail.

Fresh Air The nose, throat and lungs of a horse are very susceptible to irritation from foul air and in consequence a good airy box must be provided with efficient drainage. In comparison with the field any stable will be warm, so leave windows and top door open, otherwise sweating will occur and may result in a chill. A horse may be turned out to grass from a warm stable and, providing there is shelter from cold winds, he will seldom develop a cold or cough. On the other hand if he is brought out of a field and put into a warm badly ventilated stable invariably he will develop a cold. Of course draughts must be avoided at any time.

Feeding The sudden change from natural green foods to dry fodder is somewhat of a shock to the system and in consequence certain preparations are necessary. Hay being the nearest to grass it should form the main ingredient of the first diet. A bran mash each night will act as a slight laxative and help in the digestion of dry hay.

Diarrhoea from the sudden change of food, and fretting from being stabled, will occur for a few days but is of no consequence.

After five to six days a purgative may be given. In the past an aloes ball was used but these are much less used nowadays since if used without care or suitable preparation they can be distinctly dangerous owing to the extremely violent and possibly painful purging action especially when the bowel contains quantities of semi-dry food. This drug in its pure state is rather nauseating so that a prepared form of the same drug (Dihydroxyanthraquinone), which is tasteless and will be taken on the mash, is far preferable.

Within twelve hours this purgative will commence to work and may continue for two to three days during which time bran mashes night and morning, and a little meadow hay, should be the only feed. Naturally most animals are dull and listless during the period of purgation but such symptoms are normal and should give no cause for alarm. Accurate dosage is essential as too small a quantity will not cause purgation, resulting in the retention of the drug and considerable digestive upset. An overdose will cause excessive purgation which may be difficult to check. Purgatives may cause inflammation of the lining membrane of the bowels and on the physiological side may involve dangers which include depletion of body salts (especially potassium). In the light of these factors at the present time most people are of the opinion that this purgative is not necessary and consider a longer period of laxatives such as small doses of linseed oil, epsom salts or even castor oil, adequate.

After purgation has finished hay may be increased but a bran mash should be given twice daily for at least another week. One or two pounds of corn may be given in the mash to make it more appetising.

The maximum amount of corn to be given will depend on the size of the animal and the work to be done but the increase should be given gradually. In any case if a portion of the previous meal is left, the amount must be cut down. Corn should always be bruised as few horses will masticate whole grain.

Chaff is of value in the initial stages because, being dry, it ensures ample chewing before being swallowed.

An opinion shared by many that bran is not necessary once a horse is fit, is wrong in my opinion. A small quantity, say 1 lb. daily, is a useful adjunct to any feed at all times, used dry it helps to prevent bolting of the food, and generally acts as a laxative. Of course I am not referring to the sloppy mash that should be given each week-end as a routine. I say routine because it is so necessary to give any system a rest from large quantities of stimulating foods. Further it is essential that a bran mash be given to a horse after a hard day as so often this also means the missing of at least one meal. Fatigue results in the whole system being below par and in such a state a heavy meal will result in indigestion or maybe colic.

A little corn may be added to the mash to make it more appetising and also linseed. There is no danger in giving a little corn in the mash as it will be partly cooked with the bran.

Whilst on the subject of linseed there appears to be a considerable difference of opinion regarding the cooking of this seed, resulting in great waste, and in consequence Col. Codrington described a method which is both economical and efficient.

A breakfast cup full of linseed should be added to a gallon of cold water in an iron saucepan and allowed to simmer for at least six to eight hours. The seed has a very hard outer coating which will be toughened by placing in hot water or boiled for a short while, and this will prevent some of the nutriment in the heart of the seed from being drawn out. If cooked slowly the resultant liquid will be very thick and the seed will drop to the bottom of the saucepan. The seed can be strained off by passing the whole through a muslin cloth but this is immaterial as it will do no harm.

The quantity of jelly to be added to one mash should not exceed the amount from one breakfast cup of seed, in fact this is adequate for two horses.

A cup full of jelly may be given daily during the early preparation of a horse if it comes up in poor condition from poor keep, exposure, or excess of worms, but owing to its fatty nature it should not be continued once a horse is doing well.

The importance of a good quality hay is not appreciated to the fullest extent by many, which is a great mistake. A good class hay cut in June so that the maximum of leaf and seed is present, and carried with little or no rain, has a feeding value equivalent to corn. Hay that has had a lot of rain on it will be musty and in such a state, is most unsuitable for horses, although some may eat it with relish and leave good bright September hay because it has no seed in it.

Without going into too much detail there are two main types of hay known as Meadow and Seed or Hard Hay.

Meadow hay is made from old permanent pastures and is much softer than Seed hay. It is admirable for horses in their early preparation, when sick, for hacking, or for children's ponies, but has not the body in it that seed hay has for real hard work.

Hard or Seed Hay is made from a sown mixture of clovers, rye grass and cock's foot.

Regardless of the type hay should not be fed before December of the year it is made, but if possible should be left until the autumn of the following year.

A good quality hay should be bright yellow to green in colour, have a sweet smell, and contain a good proportion of leaf and seed. If made in July, August or September the proportion of leaf will be much lower and a great deal of seed dropped, thus reducing considerably its feeding value.

When feeding long fodder give it in a net or on the ground. If given in a high rack above the horse's head there is a danger of seeds falling into the eyes.

Oats can vary a great deal in quality and the detection of a good sample is much more simple if they are not crushed. The white oat seems to be popular today but a good sample of black or tawny has equal feeding value.

The outside husk should be shiny and the interior or heart fat. When a handful is picked up and dropped back on the bulk it should 'rattle'. When in the sack one should be able to push one's hand down into the grain easily, but if the heart is poor it is much more difficult to do so. If the grain has been badly harvested heating will have taken place and this can be detected by a musty smell. On no account should such a sample be fed as it will soon cause digestive trouble and may even affect a horse's wind.

Oats should not be fed whole as a fair proportion will pass through the gut indigested. They should be bruised, as opposed to crushed, and in a good sample the heart should be flat. Prejudice against feeding barley to horses, except in small quantities, and boiled, to put condition on a show or sick horse, has been overruled to a great extent. Ample proof of its value was obvious when fed to several thousand horses of the Cavalry Division in the Middle East in 1939, oats being unobtainable. In the case of the heavy hunter type which often develops filled legs when fed large quantities of oats, barley can be given without this effect, and with no loss in stamina. It should be bruised rather than crushed as the latter may result in a meal, which is not good for horses, and a smaller quantity is required, viz. 8 lb. of barley are equivalent to 10 lb. oats. Other advantages are:

a. It is preferable for children's ponies as it does not hot them up or affect their feet.

b. Small quantities, say 1 to 2 lb.; may be fed to sick animals that are not taking exercise with safety.

c. As it contains little or none of the anti-calcium element present in oats it has great advantages for young horses up to three years old.

Maize in a partly cooked form and known as Flaked Maize, in small quantities, may be used to put on condition but is most unsuitable for fast work.

Beans may be used in small quantities, 1½ to 2 lb. daily, the last month of a training period, but should not be given under any circumstances unless the horse is well and in full work.

Horses generally like roots especially carrots, and these are undoubtedly useful when the remainder of the diet consists of dry foods.

The orange garden variety of carrot and the white field variety are useful as an appetiser, and the latter has considerable food value, but the root that has great possibilities is the Fodder Beet. It is much more indigestible than other roots and in consequence an animal must be given a small quantity at first, say one per day, and gradually increased to a maximum of say eight a day, but their food value and suitability for horses is unquestionable. I can speak personally of hunters fed on Fodder Beet, 3 to 4 lb. of oats and a normal quantity of hay doing a long day as well as an animal fed on oats.

In conclusion may I suggest that the rations for horses should be balanced for the particular purpose that the horse is intended to serve. We should, however, not merely be content to satisfy the energy requirements but also to provide a range of foods and therefore a varied diet which will prove nutritionally adequate.

Difficult Feeders Sooner or later one is sure to come up against the animal that is not a hearty feeder but there is an answer to most of them.

Shy Feeder This is the type that is fussy about his food, and one is never quite certain when he will eat a full meal. Small quantities given more often, with the addition of a chopped carrot or green stuff, and a constant change from oats to horse cubes, or a little boiled barley will often prove successful. If possible put a shy feeder next to a good feeder; often it will act as an inducement.

Night Feeder Some horses will only pick at their food during the day but will eat up at night. The obvious answer to this problem is to give a very small quantity during the day, half a feed at evening stables, and a full feed at about 10 p.m. A horse that is inclined to bolt his food should be given small quantities more often with the addition of a little chaff which requires more mastication.

Finally remember that at least one hour should elapse between a feed and the commencement of exercise.

Watering Many theories have been propounded as to the best method of watering a horse with full reasons and in consequence I propose to deal with the subject at some length. In the natural state an animal has access to water at all times but of course his diet is not dehydrated as in a stable-fed animal.

As to whether horses should be watered before or after feeding, the rational and most satisfactory method is to follow nature and let the horse drink whenever he wants to, in which case they will not take large amounts at any one time.

Watering before food has its proponents. The argument against this method is based on the assumption that between meals gastric digestive juices are stored up to cope with the next meal, and a drink will dilute these or even flush them through the bowel. This is a false impression as the flow of digestive juices is stimulated by the sight and smell of food and its presence in the stomach.

Watering after food is suggested as being a bad principle as the digestive juices will be diluted, and solid food will be washed into the gut before due preparation. But experimental evidence has shown that when the stomach is full a copious draught of water does not mix with the stomach contents but passes straight through into the small intestine.

If a horse has free access to water he will seldom take large quantities at a time. However, there is a type that will eat a few mouthfuls of food and then have a drink and continue this procedure throughout the meal. In this case free access is not a good principle.

We can summarise the above by suggesting that regularity is the cornerstone of any watering policy and, providing that the horse has become used to the system, watering may be done before during or after a meal without interfering with digestion in any way.

Irrespective of the method adopted water should not be offered straight from a tap or well. It should be drawn and left in the stable for some time so that its temperature is the same as that of the animal's surroundings.

There is one exception to this rule. Some horses will not stale for some time after returning to the stable but if allowed just two or three mouthfuls of cold water they will usually stale at once.

If the principle of watering before meals is adopted it is advisable to leave a bucket full in the stable an hour after the last night feed.

Exercise This is important for the growth of new muscle tissue since it stimulates the formation of new fleshy material. Whilst it does this it also brings about the loss of watery and fatty material in the muscles. A general toning up of the system is also effected by exercise since the alternate contraction and relaxation of muscles exerts a pumping action on blood and lymph vessels so that fluids circulate freely. Waste products carried by them are expelled faster and the general blood supply of all tissues is increased resulting in an increased activity in heart, lungs, kidneys, liver, etc. The digestive organs are compressed and relaxed more often and more vigorously so that digestion is aided and sluggishness of the bowels or constipation is prevented. When a horse is first brought up from grass exercise is not necessary during the first week, but when purgation is over, and corn is given, work should commence.

The first week walking for half an hour is adequate and this can be increased by half an hour weekly up to the maximum of two and a half hours. Walking and trotting should be given for the first three weeks after which cantering can commence.

The advocate of three to four hours on the road or excessive fast work is wrong. As will be appreciated when dealing with leg troubles in another part of this book, it is the tired horse that develops tendon trouble and hours away from the stable, with or without long stretches of galloping, will make any horse jaded.

How often has one seen the initial states of 'a leg' appear at home through too much fast work.

In the case of a hunter doing his three days a fortnight exercise can be restricted to one and a half hours a day, except the day after hunting, when half is adequate.

As most horses stand in the stable for twenty to twenty-two hours a day a short walk in hand during the late afternoon is a welcome break from boredom and it will assist the circulation.

Clipping In view of the weakening influence of excessive sweating clipping is essential for any horse that is doing fast work. Whether the legs are left unclipped, or parts of the body, is not important, but it is advisable to leave the saddle patch. It will act as a natural protection against friction from the saddle.

Never clip a horse which is suffering from any complaint especially not a cold or other respiratory trouble, and never clip during severe weather. Give an extra ration of hay and oats to newly clipped horses to make good the loss of heat and keep the animal out of draughts for several days.

If the skin is very dirty after clipping put a couple of rugs on and give the horse a sharp canter. This will cause him to sweat and assist in cleansing the skin.

Bedding Good wheat straw is undoubtedly the best form of bedding. Oat straw may be used but is soft and will be eaten. Peat is useful when a horse eats his bedding but good drainage is essential otherwise it soon becomes sodden. Also droppings must be picked up frequently.

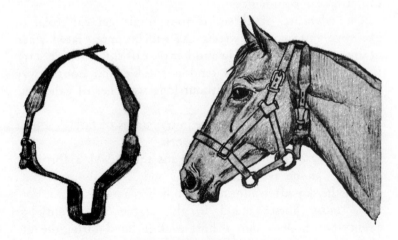

Fig. 39
left Anti-crib-biting device
right Device in position

Shavings and sawdust can be used in the same way as peat but they are cold and may cause foot trouble.

Bracken can be used but it must be dry. Green or partly withered bracken is poisonous.

To safeguard against galls it is a good plan to put a roller on from the first day. Constant movement, causing light friction, will tend to harden the skin.

Washing the Sheath Although quite important this is often overlooked. The sheath should be moistened with warm water, and a good class soap applied to form a lather to break down all the dried secretion. A liberal supply of warm water is necessary to wash off all the soap, allowed to dry, after which Vaseline should be gently massaged into the part.

VICES

Under this heading is included a group of habits or vices developed by horses due almost entirely to idleness and boredom. Once the habit has become established the animal is seldom at rest and the normal functions of the digestive and respiratory systems may be disturbed. Young horses should therefore not be left for long periods without exercise or work of some sort. It is better to turn them out to grass rather than leave them idle in a stable.

The main habits are Weaving, Wind Sucking and Crib-biting.

Weaving A horse is said to be a weaver when it sways its head and neck from side to side and at the same time lifts one leg after the other. Usually the horse is looking over a half door.

Once the habit has developed it is difficult to cure, but it can be curbed by keeping the doors closed. As the habit is prone to be copied by other horses no other animal should be allowed to see it. It may cause loss of condition and action since if constant the horse will get insufficient rest and uselessly fatigue its muscles.

Wind Sucking The horse snatches the head, as though snapping at a fly, purses the lips, arches the neck and swallows air.

Crib-biting The horse grasps the edge of a manger, arches the neck and swallows air.

Both wind sucking and crib-biting appear to be two forms of the same vice and both may cause chronic digestive trouble and colic. Crib-biting also wears the incisor teeth excessively so that in bad cases they may no longer meet when the mouth is closed rendering grazing impossible.

As the animal arches its neck before swallowing, several devices, such as a broad strap around the neck immediately behind the ears, or a metal tongue fitting under the throat, may prevent the vice, by causing pain or discomfort when the animal attempts to arch its neck. Another preventive is a hollow perforated bit which means that the horse cannot produce a vacuum in its mouth necessary for wind sucking.

An operation, whereby the muscles of the neck used in arching are cut, may cure the condition.

A further operation applicable to wind suckers involves the making of a permanent fistula from the mouth cavity. This seems to achieve good results after a brief period of accommodation during which the horse may have some difficulty swallowing.

SEQUENCE IN PREPARATION OF HORSE/PONY FROM GRASS TO HARD WORK

To some extent the following details are a repetition of those found at the beginning of this chapter but the sequence is being given in greater detail here. Quantities of food are quoted as a guide, but the table at the end of this section must be referred to for a more accurate ration.

1st to 4th day A bran mash morning and night and about 10 lb. of meadow hay. No exercise is necessary.

5th day	A dose of physic (but see the comments on the advisability of purgation in earlier chapters) on the morning mash and an ordinary mash at night. Hay 10 lb. No exercise.
6th to 9th day	A bran mash twice daily until purging has ceased, after which mashes can be cut to one daily. Hay 10 to 12 lb. No exercise.
10th to 15th day	Oats 3 lb. daily with 2 lb. of bran and a little chaff. Hay 12 lb. Exercise ½ to ¾ hour daily.
16th to 21st day	Oat or other grain 6 lb. daily with 2 lb. bran and a little chaff. Hay 15 lb. Exercise 1½ hours walking and trotting.
4th week	Oat or other grain 10 lb. daily with 1 lb. dry bran. Hard hay may now be given gradually in place of meadow hay. Exercise 2 hours. Fast work may be commenced. Fodder beet may be given now commencing with 2 a day and increased by 2 weekly up to a maximum of 6 medium sized.

If the sound practice of feeding 2 to 3 lb. of corn daily for a month prior to bringing the animal in is observed, the time of preparation can be reduced considerably. Bran mashes should be given for the first three to four days to ensure the bowel being laxative, a dose of physic given on the fifth day, and bran mashes for the next two or three days, or until purging has ceased. After this 4 to 6 lb. of corn may be given and increased by 4 lb. weekly. Hay and exercise will be the same as quoted previously according to the corn ration.

In Col Codrington's opinion, other than in exceptional circumstances, the quantity for, say, a sixteen hand middle weight horse, should never exceed 15 lb. daily.

For economical reasons many horses are kept out of doors these days, in a New Zealand Rug. In such cases the dose of physic can be dispensed with, but the corn ration must be introduced into the diet gradually. The initial ration of corn should be in the region of 3 lb. daily and increased by 4 lb. weekly. Although the animal is free to exercise itself under this system it is advisable to arrange a controlled programme according to the ration of corn given.

After hunting or any hard day's work a horse that is kept out should be housed in a cold stable, free from draught, dried with a wisp, and given a mash of 3 lb. of bran plus 3 lb. of boiled corn. By boiled corn I mean that which has been mixed with the bran before boiling water has been added to make the mash. After about one hour, by which time he should have eaten his feed and dried off, he may be turned out again.

To provide a ready reference in table form to suit all breeds and sizes would be impossible, not only because diets vary according to the individual of each type, but they must also be geared to the amount of work to be done.

The undermentioned is a rough guide to animals 14.2 h.h. and above in regular work. Should they be required to hunt 3 days a fortnight the maximum amount will be given, but if only doing 1 to 1½ hours exercise during the week and hunted on Saturday the minimum will be offered.

The successful horsemaster will know how much concentrated food each animal will eat almost to the ounce because he will check after every feed and cut down immediately should the horse not clean up. Weights are in lbs. and times can be switched as some horses eat better at some times in the day than others.

	Ingredient	14.2	Light wt. 15.2	Middle wt. 16.1	Heavy wt. 16.2 & over
8 a.m.	Oats or nuts	1	1 – 1½	1 – 2	2 – 3
	Barley	–	–	–	–
	Flaked maize	–	–	½	–
	Bran	½	½	½	½
	Beet pulp	–	½	–	–
	Hay	2	3	3	3
12	Oats or nuts	1	2 – 3	2 – 3	3 – 4
	Barley	–	½	½	1
	Bran	½	½	½	½
	Flaked maize	½	–	½	1
	Beet pulp	½	1	1	½
	Hay	3	3	3	5

5 p.m.	Oats or nuts	2	3 – 4	5 – 6	5 – 7
	Barley	1	$\frac{1}{2}$	$\frac{1}{2}$	1
	Bran	$\frac{1}{2}$	$\frac{1}{2}$	$\frac{1}{2}$	$\frac{1}{2}$
	Flaked maize	–	$\frac{1}{2}$	$\frac{1}{2}$	1
	Beet pulp	2	1	1 – 2	1 – 2
	Hay	7	9	10	12

Because most horses feed much better at night it will be noticed that the diet is proportioned at a.m. 10 per cent, noon 30 per cent, night 60 per cent.

CHAPTER SEVENTEEN

Care of Feet and Shoeing

The old adage 'No foot — no horse' is so true and many a horse has been ruined entirely from lack of attention to the feet.

Farriery is a great art which until recently appeared to by dying out owing to the diminution in the horse population. Now that the horse is promoting more interest more young men are becoming apprenticed to the trade.

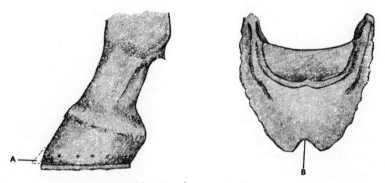

Fig. 40. Shoeing Faults

left Dumping of toe; portion rasped away shown on dotted line A
right Wasting at toe of pedal bone B, due to pressure from toe clip

To generalise, the art of shoeing can be summarised as fitting the shoe to the foot, as opposed to making the shoe and then cutting the foot to fit.

Even when at grass a foot should be attended to monthly, as one must realise that the foot is growing but the shoe remains constant.

The idea of taking all shoes off when a horse is turned out

to grass is a false economy. So often the fore feet break away badly, especially if the ground is hard, and when the time comes for shoeing it is only possible to tack a temporary shoe on until the wall grows again. Further, there is a tendency to a contracted foot afterwards. It is advisable to take the hind shoes off, especially if there are several horses together, to avoid injury from kicking.

Although the hind feet do not wear as quickly as the front it is advisable to have the feet trimmed at least once a month. Although the signs that a horse needs shoeing are fairly obvious, such as a loose shoe, raised clenches, the foot overhanging the shoe, etc., the feet should be picked up frequently to see that the branches of the shoe are not twisted and bearing on the sole, or on the seat of a corn.

Often when a horse is shod for the first time after being at grass, it will go short for a few days. Generally this is due to the shoes being put on too tight and in a day or so the action returns. Should the action not improve, or even lameness occur, it is probable that a nail is so near to the sensitive part of the foot as to cause pressure, or it has actually penetrated into the sensitive foot. In either case, each nail should be withdrawn and the shaft examined for signs of blood. If this is present, this nail should not be replaced for a day or so, but a little Tincture of Iodine forced into the hole with a syringe.

Another injury following shoeing may be brushing. The inside of the fetlock or coronet is struck by the inside of the opposite foot at the trot or canter. If severe there may be a deep wound leading to a stumble or even a fall especially if brushing occurs in front. There are many fancy shoes in use to avoid this brushing, but if the horse's action is straight, it is as well to provide bandages in the first place, as so often the cause is just weakness. This conclusion is reinforced by the observation that it is almost always found in young animals shod for the first time, old or weak animals that are overworked, out of condition animals at the beginning of the season, or tired animals at the end of a hard days work.

Shoeing A great deal has been written regarding the correct methods of shoeing but it is the interpretation that concerns us. It is a highly skilled art and one that can only be perfected by practice. However, if one has some knowledge of the structures of the foot and its functions, the initiative can and should come from the owner. Other than malpractices which have been handed down, and which can be corrected, there are certain types of shoes with which one should be familiar and demand for certain conditions.

In the past there were numerous types of shoes designed to give relief to unsound conditions, e.g. dropped soles, contracted feet, navicular disease, etc., but thanks to the vigilance of the Veterinary Profession and the R.S.P.C.A. unless a condition can be cured so that the animal recovers completely, it may not be worked. This has resulted in most of the surgical shoes being scrapped.

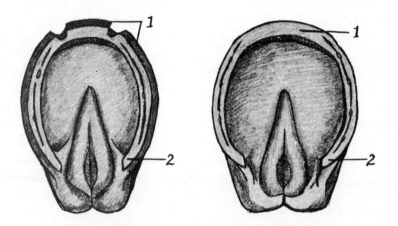

Fig. 41. Signs that shoeing is necessary
right Fore Foot
    1. Shoe worn at toe
    2. Ends of shoe bearing on sole
left Hind Foot
    1. Wall of foot showing outside shape of shoe
    2. Heels of shoe too long.

The main variations from the normal concave fullered shoes are as follows:

Tips These half-shoes are made of small light iron and cover the toe only. They are used for horses at grass, the object being to prevent the toe from being broken away and at the same time allow maximum frog pressure. They would therefore be useful during certain diseases such as contracted heels when frog pressure is necessary but would only be satisfactory for light fast work in the healthy horse.

Three Quarter Shoes In these shoes there is a deficiency on one branch of the shoe from quarters to heel intended to relieve the heel and associated structures from pressure and allow repair to occur. They are used in the case of corns, but afford no protection against stones, etc.

Feather edged Shoes These are employed to prevent brushing. The inner branch of the fore or hind shoe is made narrow to avoid it hitting the opposite limb. As brushing is often due to weakness or faulty action more specific action should be employed and will be found under the chapter on the subject.

Wedge Heeled Shoes These are used occasionally in the case of strained tendons as a temporary measure. By raising the heel the tension on the tendon is reduced during the initial stages, but it also allows the fibres of the tendon to contract. When a normal flat shoe is fitted the heel drops, resulting in renewed strain on the tendon.

Leathers Leather is sometimes employed between the foot and the shoe to minimise concussion in certain foot conditions. As a protection in the case of a bruised sole a temporary leather covering the whole sole is useful. These pads covering the entire sole should not be left on too long as dirt will work up between them and the sole and cause foot trouble. A piece of leather, the same size and shape as the shoe is used in cases of 'pottery action'. It will minimise concussion but is extremely difficult to fit.

Anti-Slipping Devices In view of the slippery state of many roads today some form of anti-slipping attachment is essential.

For ordinary hacking on the roads pads which fit across the heel are very efficient, the best known being the Gray's Pad. However, these are useless for hunting as they are soon drawn off by mud. Studs which can be either driven into the heels of the shoe or screwed are the most efficient for hunters.

The principle faults in shoeing are as follows:

1. Insufficient time and care is spent on the bearing surface of the foot to ensure it being level. The growth of horn that has occurred since the last visit to the farrier must be reduced by cutting and rasping so that the wall remains level all around the foot.
2. Excessive burning to save rasping the bed level.
3. Failing to get the angle of the toe clip the same as the wall. The clip is then hammered flat against the wall which causes pressure on the pedal bone and may result in lameness.
4. Dumping. This is the term given to the practice of rasping the wall at the toe after the shoe has been nailed on. If the shoe is fitted accurately there should be no excess of toe to be removed. The practice exists because it is compara-tively easy, and so much quicker, to knock up a shoe that more or less fits the foot, and file away any excess of horn afterwards, than to make an accurate shoe. As the portion of horn in question acts as a hold for the nails, any part of it that is filed away must weaken that hold.

In any case rasping of the wall should be discouraged as it removes the outer covering of the horn which retains the natural oil, resulting in brittle feet.

5. Rasping the clenches after they have been turned down, thereby weakening them. This should not be necessary if the wall under the nail has been recessed with the edge of the file, to accommodate the clench.

6. Cutting the bars for the purpose of opening the foot. This should not be done under any circumstances as these bars act as a reinforcement for the wall and prevent contraction of the foot.

7. Excessive paring back of the frog and sole. These structures consist of fairly brittle horn which is shed normally in flakes. Only loose or overgrown portions should be removed since it is imperative for the efficient functioning of the foot that the frog should contact the ground.

CHAPTER EIGHTEEN

Care and Management of Brood Mare and Foal

A great deal of difference of opinion exists regarding the care of a mare prior to, at, and after foaling.

Breeding is a natural process for which nature makes adequate and efficient provision. In the great majority of cases things follow a normal ordered course, a fact which is so often forgotten.

Once a mare is definitely in foal little or no harm will result if she does light work for the first six months. After this period it is advisable to cease work. Some breeders choose to bring a mare in each night, except in the height of the summer, but it is not necessary. The only advantage in so doing is that she can be under constant supervision, as most mares foal at night.

Choice of a mare. Other than a thoroughbred intended purely for racing, the choice should be governed by several basic principles:

1. **Age** Three years old is a good time, as little training can be done except long reining and backing for a short while, and in consequence the period from three to four years can be spent profitably.
2. **Conformation** A good roomy mare with bone and substance. Avoid those with faulty action and/or hereditary unsoundness in their ancestry.
3. **Temperament** This factor is so often passed on to the progeny via the dam.
4. **Constitution** As hunters and hunter chasers are under consideration staying blood is a most important factor.

It is a great mistake to mate a sprinter mare to a staying

sire or vice versa. The result is a failure more often than not.

Many people are inclined to breed from a mare that has broken down, or developed some unsoundness, or even an old favourite. Providing the fault is not in the category of hereditary unsoundness the mare may be used, but in the case of an old favourite, over fifteen years old, the progeny are often most disappointing and of poor constitution.

Mating Having chosen the mare the best time for mating is between April and June since the average gestation period is just over 11 months (340 days). This means that the foal will benefit in the early stages from the good weather and from the grass when it is at its maximum nutritional level. If the mare be mated after July the foal may arrive too late to be hardened off before the bad weather sets in.

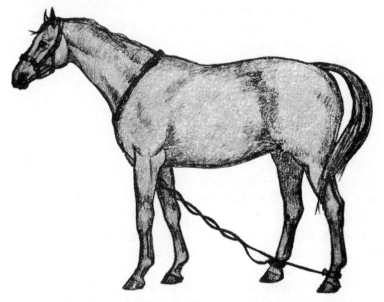

Fig. 42. Mare with service hobbles in position

The signs of a mare being in season are general slackness, and lifting of the tail, especially if the flank is handled, and passage of a small quantity of urine at the same time. If these signs are present it is justification for a visit to the stallion. When a mare is 'tried' with a stallion, if she is on heat she will not resent the horse, she will lift her tail, and the vulva will open and close, and a small quantity of mucus may be passed.

When a mare is served hobbles should be used to avoid the possibility of injury to the stallion. If the simple 'service hobble' is used the horse cannot get entangled in the rope and the mare can move enough to avoid falling down. After service the mare should be walked about for at least twenty to thirty minutes.

After service the mare should be 'tried' with the horse at three weeks and six weeks in case she has turned. Occasionally a mare will 'take the horse' even though she be in foal, also a mare may not show heat and not be in foal.

From fifty to ninety days after service the blood can be tested and after seventeen weeks the urine, to determine if the mare is in foal. These tests are carried out if samples are sent by a Veterinary Surgeon to the Equine Research Station, Newmarket. As these tests are quite reliable, it is an obvious economy to have them done. A further sign of pregnancy will be a general change in temperament, i.e. they become more docile. If viewed from behind there is an increase in the size of the stomach, the underneath of which appears to be flat. At about the seventh month movement of the foal may be seen or felt in the flank, especially after a drink of cold water.

Foaling Taking everything into consideration it is perhaps the wisest plan to foal a mare in the stable so that help may be at hand in case of complications. From the point of view of disease or injury, if a suitable field is available and handy, and the weather is good, many people think this method is preferable.

If the mare is to be foaled in the stable a good big roomy box should be chosen and she should be brought in each night for at least two to three weeks prior to the foaling date to get her used to the box. A light should be provided and left on each night and a hole provided in the wall or partition so that the mare can be watched, especially at foaling time, without disturbing her. This is most important as so often the presence of an attendant, even if known to the mare, will put her off.

Corn should be given throughout pregnancy, and a daily mash the last week to keep the bowels lax and overcome the usual constipation.

The hind shoes should be removed before foaling to avoid injury to the foal.

The signs that a mare is very close to foaling are:

a. Rapid development of the udder;

b. Dropping of the muscles on either side of the root of the tail;

c. Swelling of the vulva;

d. A small droplet of yellow waxy material develops on the end of the teats;

e. In the field the mare is invariably away on her own, often in a corner.

The immediate signs of foaling are:

a. Running of milk;

b. Restlessness;

c. Kicking at the stomach;

d. Swishing of the tail;

e. Very enlarged and slack vulva;

f. Getting up and down;

g. Finally, actual labour pains occur.

The actual act of foaling is usually very rapid. Often it is completed in not more than twenty minutes from the onset of labour. Should it be longer, it must be assumed that there is something wrong with the presentation of the foal and professional advice should be sought at once.

Sometimes with a normal presentation the head and fore legs are out but the foal is held at the hips, in which case assistance must be given. Also a foal is sometimes born with the after-birth over the nostrils and if that is not removed at once the foal may be suffocated. After removal make certain that the foal is breathing and, if not, artificial respiration should be given. The upper fore leg should be lifted up and down and at the same time, with each downward movement gentle pressure should be applied to the ribs with the palm of the hand. A foal may be injured if the pressure be too severe. Once the foal is breathing normally the next step was always stipulated as being to tie and cut the navel cord. However, recent work at the Equine Research Station at Newmarket has suggested that the umbilical cord is best not interfered with since too early a separation may deprive the newborn foal of up to 1½ litres of blood contained within the placenta (afterbirth). If the cord is allowed to break naturally, and there is a point at which rupture is easily accomplished, the amount of blood lost (remaining in the afterbirth) is much less. Therefore it is suggested that the navel cord requires no human attention provided that it is allowed to break at the correct place and time generally by the mare getting up. There is normally no haemmorhage risk from the stump and less risk of infection than if the cord is cut with scissors. The tying off of the cord with tape is undesirable especially if the tape is treated with iodine since this strong antiseptic is destructive to such delicate tissues. If the mare is lying down, let her remain so for at least half an hour, but as a rule she will get up immediately after foaling. As the mare's licking is the best method of drying the foal, a little salt sprinkled over the foal will act as an inducement.

The foal, after many attempts, is usually on its feet within the hour and some may find their way to the teat, whereas others, either from weakness or other cause, will need help. It is advisable to have the mare's head held, and an attendant should push on the foal's hind quarters whilst you steer the head to the udder, place your finger in the foal's mouth (invariably they will suck), and guide the mouth to the teat, squeeze the latter with the free fingers and after some time, and a great deal of patience, one is usually rewarded.

The next worry may be that the mare has not passed the

afterbirth. As mares are particularly susceptible to blood poisoning from retained foetal membranes, should they not be voided within four hours, professional aid must be called to remove them.

A hot mash should be given to the mare after foaling. If she does not take to her foal at once an attendant should be present when the foal is sucking and, for a day or two, after each feed, the foal should be put behind some barrier, such as a gate across a corner of the box, until the mare accepts her new responsibility.

The only other immediate anxiety is that the foal must pass a motion within a few hours after birth. It is most important that the 'foetal dung' be expelled and, if the foal is seen to strain without result, an enema of warm soap and water, to which a little olive oil has been added, should be given. Two tablespoons of castor oil should be administered per mouth.

After three to four days, providing the weather is reasonable, the mare and foal should be put out for an hour the first day. Subsequently the time can be increased daily.

If the mare is to be bred from again she should be tried any time from the seventh to the eleventh day after foaling.

Should the mare be taken some distance to the stallion, she may sweat from excitement at being parted from the foal. If this happens, the mare should cool down on returning before the foal sucks, otherwise the foal may scour.

When the foal is weaned, at about seven months, either it can be done gradually by allowing it to suck less each day, or it can be done at once. In the latter case, if the mare has a lot of milk, a little may have to be drawn off daily for a week or so and the udder wiped over daily with vinegar. Green foods should not be given during this drying off period. Once the foal has been taken away it is advisable to avoid the possibility of the mare seeing it, otherwise this can cause a flushing of milk.

In the case of a colt that is not required for breeding, it is usually castrated as a yearling. Generally this operation is performed during May, or early June, but where a colt does not develop a good neck, it is wise to defer the event, even as late as September, as by so doing, often the neck will develop.

It is advisable to withhold food for at least twelve hours before the operation to avoid unnecessary risks. In the event of casting it is safer to do so on an empty stomach. A further advantage of fasting is that if the animal is turned out directly after it will commence to feed and so forget the operation.

Castration should not be performed if there is an East wind as most colts sweat during the operation and if turned out in this state are much more susceptible to chill.

Tetanus or lock jaw is another risk but this can be avoided by the injection of anti-tetanic serum prior to the operation.

DISEASES OF FOALS

Constipation Normally a substance called colostrum is present in the first milk and acts as a purgative to the foal and ensures the evacuation of the foetal dung. Should this not occur, the foal is soon dull and listless, gets up and down, shows colicky pains and strains frequently. A dose of castor oil, about two to three tablespoons, should be given by the mouth, followed by an enema of warm soapy water, to which a little olive oil has been added. Occasionally, it may be necessary to remove the first hard pellets in the rectum with the fingers.

Diarrhoea This can occur in a foal from indigestion from excessive milk, or nibbling at bedding. A dose of milk of magnesia, 2 tablespoons daily for three days, will generally clear it up, *but* if the diarrhoea is coupled with a rise in temperature, *professional advice must be sought at once,* as the cause may be due to an infection which needs speedy treatment.

Naval Ill (Joint Ill) This is due to an infection which gains access to the blood usually through the navel. The main symptoms occur at about the fifth to seventh day, the foal being listless, lying down a great deal, and the temperature rising several degrees. There may be diarrhoea and an increased rate of breathing. One or several joints becomes swollen, hot and painful to the touch and an abcess may form which bursts.

Treatment Prevention is the main consideration in dealing with this disease. Absolute cleanliness and rigid disinfection of all foaling boxes should be carried out before and after each mare has foaled. Where climatic and other conditions are favourable the dam should be allowed to foal out of doors. For mares an open or partly open shed in the corner of a sheltered paddock would fit the bill.

Severance of the navel cord is best left to the mare, and strong disinfectants should not be applied to the stump. If the cord is required to be cut the strictest personal cleanliness must be observed, and the application of a sulphanilamide dry dressing is safer than iodine solution.

Treatment with antibiotics may effect a cure and is worth trying, but so often the damage to the joints in an established case is so extensive that the animal does not regain normal action.

Preventive measures should be aimed at not interfering with the umbilical cord and ensuring as far as possible that the foal obtains a full supply of colostrum. The mother during life will have contacted most of the germs concerned and will presumably have developed antibodies to counteract their effects. These antibodies are highly concentrated in the colostrum and serve as a strong protection for the foal during the first weeks of life. Foals deprived of colostrum are more susceptible to joint-ill. This deprivation may result from the dam 'running milk' for some time prior to foaling. Should this occur the newborn foal should receive antibiotic treatment from the moment of birth.

Sleepy Foal Disease This is a disease named from its main symptom of extreme dullness. It is caused by a germ contracted from the dam. The foal is usually weakly and dies within two to three days.

Treatment with streptomycin may effect a cure if used in time, but the onset of symptoms is so rapid that by the time a diagnosis is made it is often too late.

Foal Jaundice This condition is not due to a germ, but to an incompatibility of the blood of the mare and sire.

The mechanism leading to the disease in foals has many similarities to the condition in humans associated with the rhesus factor of human blood.

The mare has substances in her first milk which destroy the red cells of the blood of the foal. There is no sign of a temperature, but within a day or so, the foal appears very listless and shortly after, the eyes, nostrils and mouth become yellow, and a dark brown urine is passed.

Treatment Recently blood transfusions have effected cures, but prevention is the main line of attack. Your Veterinary Surgeon can have samples of blood from the sire and dam examined and grouped before service to avoid the condition occurring at the next foaling.

Foal Pneumonia Recently the Equine Research Station of the Animal Health Trust have discovered the germ which causes this type of pneumonia characterised by abscess in the lungs.

Treatment This is not efficient and inclined to be speculative but once your Veterinary Surgeon has diagnosed the condition he will take the necessary steps to avoid the spread of this infection to other foals.

Before terminating the discussion on Foal diseases let us consider certain actual deformities. Occasionally a foal is born that is unable to straighten the limb or limbs below the fetlock, the result being that the animal walks on the front of the fetlock joint. In most cases the joint can be straightened, but on moving, the foal appears to have no control of the part and knuckles over immediately. It would appear that the extensor tendon in front of the leg, which keeps the toe forward, does not function.

Treatment If artificial support is given to the limb from the fetlock downwards, in the form of a plaster of paris bandage, or a leather or piroplastic legging, for about two weeks, and the leg is kept set in the normal position, the condition will often resolve.

Before applying the plaster of paris a good padding of cotton wool should be wrapped around the leg, otherwise the plaster should be taken off at the end of a week and replaced if necessary. If chafing has occurred in the front of the joint a liberal supply of sulphanilamide powder should be applied to the area before replacing the bandage.

CHAPTER NINETEEN

Heredity

In discussing this subject one must bear in mind the adage 'exception proves the rule', but there is sufficient evidence that certain characteristics and abnormal conditions are handed down through the male or female line. On such evidence does the choice of dam and sire depend.

With regard to characteristics it was Col. Codrington's opinion that:

>Temperament follows the female line
>Staying power follows the male line
>Speed follows the male line
>Jumping follows the female line
>Constitution follows the female line

When considering abnormal conditions they may not be handed down to progeny as such but the predisposition is. As an example, because a mare suffers from ringbone it does not follow that all her progeny will develop ringbone, but it is quite probable that they will be susceptible to bone disease of any type, e.g. sesamoiditis, navicular disease, etc.

Either in male or female the main unsound conditions to be avoided are:

In wind   Whistling, roaring, emphysema.
Bone   Ringbone, navicular disease, persistent splints.
Nervous origin Shivering, stringhalt.
Conformation Lack of bone, weak tendons, sloping pasterns, sickle hocks.

The above are obviously a generalisation as frequently it is a problem to decide the actual cause of an animal developing an unsoundness of wind and limb.

Some horses have been known to develop a whistle

immediately after a very hard race, whilst others have made a noise through being worked too soon after a cold, especially one following a sea journey. Such cases appear to have an obvious origin but as all are not affected the question of predisposition arises. There is also the case of the show jumper who so often develops wind trouble after three or four seasons. It is quite possible that such a defect may be caused through the sudden concerted effort required of such an animal together with lack of adequate conditioning.

It may be due to tension of the nerves which activate the muscles of the larynx or the effect of toxins or poisons elaborated at some previous illness such as strangles.

However, the fact remains that it is not a wise plan to breed from a mare that is unsound of her wind if it can be avoided.

In the case of bone diseases such as ringbone, navicular disease, and spavin, either may be brought on by excessive work or sudden strain. This applies especially to spavin, the polo pony who uses his hocks more than most being the most susceptible. The common bred horse is more susceptible to bone diseases which might be explained by the fact that the bone of such animals is coarse and weak and therefore more liable to concussion from fast work.

Again only a proportion of animals suffer from these defects and this fact points to an hereditary predisposition.

Weakness in conformation such as lack of bone, weak tendons, sickle hocks, sloping pasterns should be avoided if possible in any brood mare, and lastly shivering and stringhalt at all cost.

In conclusion it must be pointed out that a certain amount of work has been done by some eminent members of the Veterinary Profession linking unsoundness of wind and bone diseases with faulty dietetics. There is evidence that there is a connection but it is not sufficiently conclusive to quote at this juncture.

CHAPTER TWENTY

Care and Management of Sick Animals

The nursing of any sick animal will depend on the specific malady, but in general should be aimed at assisting the normal repair processes of Nature whilst in no way hindering them. A seriously ill animal requires all its strength to enable it to fight against disease and every little source of irritation acts unfavourably. We can therefore suggest several general principles under the following headings in this order:

1. Cleanliness – of patient, attendant, loose-box, bedding, etc.;
2. Comfort – light airy box, good dry bed, warmth and grooming;
3. Diet – soft easily digested yet concentrated diet and a liberal supply of fresh water;
4. Relief of pain – by appropriate treatment.

Cleanliness The fact that sick animals may discharge purulent infective material means that stable hygiene is of paramount importance. Hands and arms should be washed in antiseptic before and after attending the sick. All bedding, food, water, in fact everything coming in contact with the sick animal must be as clean as possible. Don't forget either that it takes very little trouble to sponge eyes, nostrils or the genitals with a weak antiseptic solution, the freshening effect alone of this will be of great value.

Comfort A good airy box should be provided with efficient drainage and a thick dry bed. Because fresh air is essential in combating disease, should the animal require warmth, supply it in the form of clothing — rugs, bandages, hood. Do not shut windows and doors at any time, but do not expose the animal to draughts. This applies particularly to colds, coughs and lung diseases.

As to bedding, if the ailment concerns the limbs, causing pain in movement, e.g. Lymphangitis, the straw should be cut up — a sheaf cut in at least three. If the straw is long it may become entangled around the feet and throw the animal down.

A box with a strong beam overhead may be necessary where slings are required. In the cases where the horse is down an especially thick straw bed will be necessary and the horse should be turned onto the other side two or three times a day.

Light grooming will always help, as it will promote circulation and thereby assist in eliminating any poisons. In any case remove rugs and bandages at least twice a day and give a good shaking. Light hand massage to limbs and shoulders under the roller will be beneficial.

Diet Generally speaking, the object in combating disease is the conservation of energy to fight the condition. In consequence, food must be selected for its digestibility value, and, of course, palatability. Bran mashes and green foods are always useful, as they are nourishing, slightly laxative to aid elimination, and easily digested. Milk and eggs may be added to the mash and a little boiled corn may be given as an appetiser. Rich seed hay, barley, peas and beans should always be avoided in sickness, as they are too indigestible. A liberal supply of water must be given at all times. As this is most important try and avoid giving medicines in the water that have any taste and might put the animal off drinking.

In any event offer small feeds and often, and when giving bran mashes always add a little salt, as it will make them more appetising. Sometimes some freshly cut carrots, potatoes or apples spread on top of the mash will induce a sick horse to eat.

When one is trying to persuade an animal to eat, if taken into a field it will sometimes pick a little grass, whereas it would not eat it cut and given in the stable.

Where there is difficulty in swallowing, sloppy mashes, linseed tea, eggs and milk, and steamed hay should be offered.

Because food and water soon become contaminated from nasal discharge, both should be replenished frequently when such a condition exists.

Treatment One cannot discuss this in detail here, but merely generalise.

Infections of Nose, Throat and Lungs Do not drench as the throat may be sore and there is a danger of the liquid going into the lungs. Medicines if possible should be mixed with glycerine, or treacle and flour, to make a paste, and smeared on the tongue and teeth.

Inhalations of volatile drugs by means of steamed hay will be found beneficial.

Swollen limbs from injury – abscess formation or lymphangitis require fomentation. The water should not be hotter than one can stand oneself and, to increase the drawing properties, a handful of epsom salts should be added to each bucketful.

A large piece of blanket is most useful for fomenting, as it will retain heat longer. When fomentations are finished, where possible, the part should be covered to retain the heat – even poulticed. There is one important point to remember in applying poultices. Some material impervious to moisture, such as mackintosh, greaseproof paper, and oiled silk, must be applied over the poultice. If this is not done the poultice material will draw its moisture from the atmosphere instead of from the tissue.

General inflammation from bruising, such as broken knees, or sprains to tendons, may be reduced after the intial treatment of heat, by cold hosing. By far the best results will be obtained by applying a running hose for twenty minutes at a time two or three times a day, rather than for an hour at a time. A combination of these two methods is in common usage, i.e., alternate warm and cold applications.

If the temperature rises following an injury this indicates that infection has occurred. *A veterinary surgeon should be called to apply more specific treatment.*

Method of taking a temperature

1. Before commencing shake the thermometer down until it reads below 100° F. (37.4° C.).
2. Grease with a little Vaseline, insert at least two-thirds into rectum and hold there for a full minute. If not held it may be drawn into the rectum and be difficult to recover.
3. Rinse or wash in cold water. A clinical thermometer only registers up to 110° F. so will burst if washed in hot water.
4. As infection could be carried from one animal to another by a thermometer it should be immersed in a cold solution of disinfectant after use.

First Aid Remedies

Hot Fomentations Unless one is prepared to apply such treatment for at least half an hour at a time it will have little value. The water should not be hotter than one can immerse one's hands in and a kettle of boiling water should be at hand to add to the bucket as it cools. An old piece of thick cloth such as a blanket should be used as it will hold the heat longer than a thin material. The addition. of a handful of epsom salts will increase the drawing properties of the water.

Cold Hosing This method of treatment to reduce inflammation is valuable in some cases. Running water should be used and the maximum effect will be gained if applied for twenty minutes at a stretch several times a day rather than for a longer period less frequently. It is advisable to grease the heels well before commencing to avoid soreness.

Wound Dressings: Primary in the field. Apply dry salt, sugar or epsom salts if there is no appreciable bleeding, and cover with a rag or bandage where possible. If the wound is in the foot iodine may be used.
Secondary On returning to the stable wash the wound well with plenty of hot water to which salt or epsom salts has been added – a handful to a bucket of water.

If it is only a surface would and does not need stitching dust twice daily with proflavine or sulphonamide powder. Once a scab has formed do not remove it as it is a natural covering.

If a wound needs stitching a dry dressing only should follow as watery applications will weaken the stiches.

Punctured wounds should be poulticed.

Poultice The following materials may be used:

Bran	most useful for feet.
Kaolin	the most efficient where no wound accompanies the inflammation.
Epsom salts and glycerine	made into a thick paste is beneficial in case of punctured wounds.
Moist brewer's yeast	invaluable in cases where deep seated infection needs to be drawn out.

When the poultice can be bandaged on to the part it must be covered with some material impervious to water, viz. mackintosh, oiled silk or thick greaseproof paper.

Antiseptics As an initial dressing any reputable non-irritant antiseptic may be used, e.g. Dettol, to overcome gross infection from dirt, but, as explained in detail under wound treatment, most antiseptics have been largely superseded by antibiotics for subsequent treatment.

Cough Paste (Electuary) These may be divided into two forms.
1. One containing a drug that will soothe the throat such as Potassium chlorate, Friar's Balsam, Camphor.
2. One containing a medicament that will check infection of the glands of the throat, such as sulphonamide.

The basis of either is glycerine and/or black treacle or honey, and linseed meal to thicken to a paste.

Inhalations Force a quantity of hay into a bucket and put into a sack. Pour a kettle of boiling water over the hay and sprinkle either Eucalyptus, Friar's Balsam or Menthol on the latter. Hold the mouth of the sack around the horse's nose.

Cooling Lotions

Zinc Sulphate	1 ounce
Lead Acetate	1 ounce
Rain water	1½ pints

Sprinkle a little on the part or on a piece of lint and keep in position with a bandage where possible. Re-moisten lint every four hours.

Cooling Paste
      Ceiling white
      White wine vinegar   made into a paste.
Spread on a piece of lint one-eighth of an inch thick, apply to part and bandage lightly. Renew every twelve hourse. Only make sufficient for one application at a time as its beneficial effect is soon lost when mixed.

Anodyne Paste
     1. Tincture of Arnica   1 part
        Glycerine   2 parts
     2. Adrenaline paste

Stimulating Liniments
Most of these are a mixture of ammonia and/or camphor in oil, but are irritant and cannot be used for any length of time without causing irritation. On the other hand Methylated Soap Liniment is very effective and can be used for a much longer period.

Stimulating Drench
     1. Sal Volatile   1 ounce
        Cold water   1 pint
     2. Glucose   ½ lb.
        Water   1½ pints

Purgative [Remember the warnings stated in earlier chapters about the possible ill-effects of purgation]
     1. Istin. Dose prescribed by a Veterinary Surgeon.
This is a form of aloes rendered less nauseating and tasteless. It is very efficient but the dosage must be accurate.

     2. Linseed Oil   1 pint

This may be given as one dose but should not be repeated as the horse is susceptible to an overdose.

Electrical Therapy

Much has been written concerning the value or otherwise of electrical treatment and some of the claims are no doubt genuine, but a great deal of work needs to be done before any specific effect can be substantiated.

In any case the absorption of rays is considerably lessened by deflection from hair and in consequence the effect cannot be compared with that in humans.

The main treatments under this heading are:

Infra Red rays There is little evidence that this type of ray has any specific effect except that of producing surface heat and relief of superficial pain.

Where unctions are required to have some effect on tissues under the skin their penetration is assisted by the action of the ray in dilating the skin pores.

In the case of bony outgrowths such as ringbone, sore shins, and spavins, iodine is claimed to have the power of absorbing this additional bone. A paste containing a 10 per cent iodine in a base of horse fat applied to a bone outgrowth and followed up with ten to fifteen minutes of infra red rays has proved beneficial. This treatment needs to be continued daily for at least three to four weeks.

The difference between this and heat application through poultices is that it is dry and not moist heat. Poulticing also means that heat is applied at a high temperature but quickly dissipates. Infra red treatment means that the temperature is raised slowly and can be maintained at a steady temperature for as long as desired.

Ultra Violet Rays It has been proved that these rays do have a specific effect on certain skin diseases including ringworm, alopecia (baldness) and certain forms of eczema, but their main effect is in the treatment of rickets. The results, however, are not so marked in animals as in humans because of the presence of hair, and the fact that the rays are unable to penetrate any great distance. Benefit often follows a course of irradiation in cases of localized grease and psoriasis.

Short Wave Therapy The principles of this treatment are quite different from any ray treatment in that they depend on radio waves. The actual machine emits radio waves which have the effect of penetrating all living tissue. There are two pads which are placed on either side of a mass of tissue; waves pass from each pad through the tissue in the form of an arc and where they meet heat is produced. According to the positioning of these pads a stimulant action and heat can be produced at almost any depth of tissue which of course gives it great advantages over massage and ray lamps whose action is mostly surface.

Being able to pinpoint a deep seated area such as the shoulder or hip gives this method of treatment obvious advantages over any other.

In horses with flexor tendon trouble 20 minute treatments over a period of a week are considered more effective than the old blistering and firing techniques. Consequently the most satisfactory results have been obtained in the treatment of sprained tendons, ligaments and joints and especially the sub-acute types after the initial acute inflammatory symptoms have subsided.

Electrotherapy or Faradism. This is a method of electrical treatment which may be useful for treating strains, sprains, contusions, and cases of muscular paralysis and consequent atrophy. It has been used as a standard physiotherapeutical treatment in humans for many years. The method of treatment is based upon the application of an electric current to the muscles to produce rhythmic muscle contractions which exercise the muscle without actually moving the parts. In cases of tendon strain we mentioned earlier that some degree of exercise was required to prevent adhesions from occurring. As a result of the contraction and relaxation with its attendant chemical and circulatory changes the normal physiological contraction of muscle is simulated but without producing pain. This promotes increased blood supply but it also prevents stagnation by muscular movement. Daily treatments of 20 minutes or so after the acute inflammatory stage has passed will often prove beneficial.

APPENDIX

Glossary

Back at the Knee The anterior line of the leg is concave and the posterior line tends to be convex at the knee.

Bold Eye A prominent eye. Denotes a bold character.

Bold Front Good length of neck, well muscled with good head carriage. Generally denotes a horse with courage.

Bone Refers to the span of bone and tendons just below the knee.

Closely coupled A short back and well ribbed up.

Cresty Thick convex neck as seen in stallions. Causes lack of flexibility.

Daisy Cutter Refers to rather extravagant extension of the fore legs when trotting with the feet only just clearing the ground. Denotes good shoulder movement covering plenty of ground at each stride.

Dipped Back (Swamped Back) A hollow back. Although often a good ride, as the weight of the rider is carried on the back such an animal tires quickly.

Dish face A concave line of face. No detriment; may be a sign of Arab ancestry.

Ewe Neck The top line of the neck is concave. A bad carriage of the head is the result, causing difficulty in flexion.

Good bone Viewed from the side it refers to a good flat span. Capable of carrying weight as far as the bone is concerned, and strong tendons.

Goose rumped An exaggerated slope from the jumping bump to the root of the tail. No detriment except from the look. Often a good jumper.

215

Heavy fronted Wide chest and very muscular. Denotes lack of quality and often a bad mover.

Heavy topped Heavy muscular body out of proportion to the limbs. Such lack of proportion predisposes to leg strain.

Herring gutted No depth of stomach. Denotes poor doers.

High action or climbing Extravagant movement of the fore and hind legs when galloping, lifting the body too far off the ground. This extra action must shorten the distance covered by each stride and the extra effort tires a horse quicker.

Knee action Spoken of when a horse flexes and lifts his knee well off the ground, usually seen in hackneys. This action must shorten the stride and is usually a poor ride.

Loaded shoulder Thick muscular shoulder and withers not prominent. A horse with this fault is generally a poor mover and often rolls in his trot and gallop.

Narrow in front Little space between the fore legs. Besides denoting a restricted space for heart and lungs, such a fault predisposes to brushing.

Over at the Knee The anterior line of the leg is markedly convex at the knee.

Parrot mouth The teeth of the lower jaw are set behind those of the upper jaw. A disadvantage to the animal as it will be unable to bite off short grass.

Peacocky High head carriage, upright of shoulder. No detriment in itself but often goes with narrow, flighty horses.

Pig eye An eye that is sunken and small. Often means a mean character.

Pigeon toed The fore feet turn in. No detriment at all.

Pin toed The fore feet turn out. A distinct fault as it predisposes to brushing, and such animals are poor movers in deep going.

Ragged hips Hip points prominent and far apart.

Roman nose Viewed from the side the line of the face is convex. Although denoting lack of quality, it often signifies a good sensible horse and honest worker.

Showing wear Refers to fetlock joints that are rounded and thickened owing to work. (Apple joints.)

Slab sided Ribs that are flat as opposed to well rounded. A flat rib means a restricted chest space and heart room.

Slack of a rib A large space between the last rib and the point of the hip. This denotes a long back and thus a weakness.

Throaty Coarse behind the lower jaw and bottom line of the neck. Shows lack of quality but no detriment.

Tied in below the knee Refers to a weak cannon and tendons. Unable to carry weight.

Well let down Long well-sprung ribs, long forearm and second thigh, and short cannon bone. Denotes good space of chest to accommodate heart and lungs, and a good mover because of the longer forearm and second thigh.

Well ribbed up A small space between the last rib and the point of the hip. This goes with a short back and denotes strength.

Well sprung ribs The reverse of slab sided.

Index

Warts, 134
Weaving, 179
Whistling, 128
Wind: whistling and roaring, 128
Withers, fistulous, 163
Worms, 109; red, 113; seat, 110
Wounds, 51: general treatment of, 52;
  broken knees, 59; over-reach, 57;
  punctured, 55; thorn, 60